Me, Myself & My Multiple Myeloma

PRAISE FOR *ME, MYSELF & MY MULTIPLE MYELOMA*

Praise for Ray Hartjen's poignancy, openness, and generosity in sharing his cancer experience with us. I was immediately captivated and appreciative of his practical suggestions. Congratulations, Ray, on an inspirational book!

Sandra J. Wing, founder & executive director, Sandra J. Wing Healing Therapies Foundation

More than 20,000 men and women are diagnosed annually with the incurable blood cancer called multiple myeloma. But only Ray Hartjen has the eloquence to describe its harsh realities while patiently escorting the reader, step-by-step, through the life-extending therapies that, for lucky patients like him, make this insidious disease manageable for years, even decades, to come. Written in easy-to-understand prose, this multiple myeloma memoir brings you the latest facts, insightful tips, occasional wit, and deeply reassuring advice. In addition to the book's honesty, there is a genuine humanity, a kindness, within the pages. For these reasons, *Me, Myself & My Multiple Myeloma* is a must-read for every patient and their caregivers.

Fran Carpentier, publishing and media strategist

Me, Myself & My Multiple Myeloma is an inspiring book and a must-read for anyone who is not just curious as a patient, caregiver, or a family member dealing with a multiple myeloma diagnosis. It's also a roadmap to living life to its fullest with all of its sunrises and sunsets.

Irene Lerner, educator and lifelong learner

Me, Myself & My Multiple Myeloma is more than just a guide to living with multiple myeloma. It is a testament to the courage, resilience, and hope of the author, who shares his personal journey and insights with honesty and compassion. Anyone who is affected by this condition, whether as a patient, a family member, a caregiver, or a friend, will find inspiration and support in these pages. I highly recommend *Me, Myself & My Multiple Myeloma* to anyone who wants to learn more about multiple myeloma and how to cope with its challenges.

Brian L. Thomas, cofounder of Prosperity Toolkit, Intentional Living coach, author, and speaker

If you or a loved one ever has to face multiple myeloma, *Me, Myself & My Multiple Myeloma* is the book for you! Ray Hartjen pulls back the curtain on the highs and lows of his fight and leaves you informed and inspired by his personal vulnerability, humor, and pragmatic yet positive spirit.

Denise Lee Yohn, author of *What Great Brands Do* and *FUSION*

Me, Myself & My Multiple Myeloma details the author's incredible journey battling the physical and mental challenges of being diagnosed with an incurable disease. *Me, Myself & My Multiple Myeloma* is both inspirational and motivating—a must-read for all! Having witnessed Ray's journey, his zest for life, and his desire to help others—regardless of how he is feeling—has been remarkable. Perhaps we all need a new slogan . . . "Be like Ray."

Tom O'Lenic, biotechnology executive and author

ME, MYSELF & MY MULTIPLE MYELOMA

A Behind-the-Scenes Look for Patients, Caregivers & Allies

RAY HARTJEN

NEW YORK

LONDON • NASHVILLE • MELBOURNE • VANCOUVER

Me, Myself & My Multiple Myeloma

A Behind-the-Scenes Look for Patients, Caregivers & Allies

Published in New York, New York, by Morgan James Publishing. Morgan James is a trademark of Morgan James, LLC. www.MorganJamesPublishing.com

Proudly distributed by Publishers Group West®

Scriptures marked KJV are taken from the KING JAMES VERSION (KJV): KING JAMES VERSION, public domain.

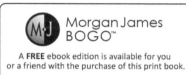

Morgan James BOGO™

A **FREE** ebook edition is available for you or a friend with the purchase of this print book.

CLEARLY SIGN YOUR NAME ABOVE

Instructions to claim your free ebook edition:
1. Visit MorganJamesBOGO.com
2. Sign your name CLEARLY in the space above
3. Complete the form and submit a photo of this entire page
4. You or your friend can download the ebook to your preferred device

ISBN 9781636983349 paperback
ISBN 9781636983356 ebook
Library of Congress Control Number:
2023947147

Cover & Interior Design by:
Christopher Kirk
www.GFSstudio.com

Front Cover Photography by:
Herb Real
Birkdale Creatives

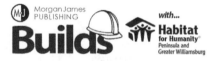

Morgan James PUBLISHING Builds with... Habitat for Humanity Peninsula and Greater Williamsburg

Morgan James is a proud partner of Habitat for Humanity Peninsula and Greater Williamsburg. Partners in building since 2006.

Get involved today! Visit: www.morgan-james-publishing.com/giving-back

To my loving and supportive wife, Lori, my two children, Olivia and Raymond, my extended family, and my network of friends and coworkers—my team—who have been so generous with their love and compassion over the years.
Most importantly, this book is dedicated to those courageous warriors: cancer patients, cancer patient medical providers, and the most unsung heroes of them all, cancer patient caregivers.
You inspire me each and every day.

TABLE OF CONTENTS

Foreword xi

Chapter 1 | D-Day 1
Chapter 2 | Say It Ain't So 11
Chapter 3 | Getting into the Fight 21
Chapter 4 | A Process, Not an Event 29
Chapter 5 | He Said, She Said 39
Chapter 6 | To Weed or Not to Weed, That Is the Question 49
Chapter 7 | Hair Today, Gone Tomorrow. 63
Chapter 8 | The First Steps of the Stem Cell Transplant Journey . . . 69
Chapter 9 | Dealing With Chemotherapy-Induced Nausea 93
Chapter 10 | The Second Half of the Stem Cell Transplant:
              Preparative Regimen, Transplant
              & Recovery. 101
Chapter 11 | The Indefatigable Human Spirit
              (and Hello Kitty Too!). 125
Chapter 12 | Who's Buried in Taken for Granted's Tomb? 135
Chapter 13 | Taking the Steps to Physical Recovery,
              One at a Time. 143

Chapter 14 | A Different Slant on Being Disabled 157
Chapter 15 | Scanxiety. 163
Chapter 16 | Perception and a New Reality 175
Chapter 17 | That Terminal Condition We Call "Life" 185

Conclusion | Next Steps 193
Acknowledgments 197
About the Writer 201
Endnotes. 203

FOREWORD

I t was a sinking feeling dropping into the pit of my gut, pervading every thought and feeling with uneasiness and uncertainty. Just seconds earlier had come, "I am so sorry."

The three words that preempted my life changing forever. What followed from an unfamiliar voice on the other end of the line was straightforward and gutting.

"You have lymphoma."

I knew little about that word—just enough to understand that I had cancer. And the diagnosis came so abruptly from a doctor I barely knew who broke the news on a phone call.

Immediately, my head, and those of my husband and our families, began swimming in questions: What are we going to do? What's next? Where do we go? How are our lives going to change?

And for me, the hardest-hitting one: Am I going to die?

The first images my mind conjured as I sat clutching my phone, feeling numb and blank, were those from the movies. Bald head, pale face, IV pole—maybe a love story sandwiched between—and then death. Was that going to be my story? My ending?

In a race for answers to gain some sense of control, my husband reached out to a childhood friend of his, a medical doctor practicing at the University of California San Francisco (UCSF), who was in our living room nearly an hour later. David's presence lifted some of that weight that had sunken us all into a dark place. Though not a medical oncologist, he helped walk us through the next steps of what might happen and what our options were.

That was what we needed right then. To be told in human terms, not in medical jargon, what this diagnosis meant on a larger scale and how we could move forward. For instance, he suggested that since we had a preliminary diagnosis, we should go to the Emergency Department at UCSF instead of trying to book an oncology appointment, which could take a lot of time. It worked, and I was immediately in the system getting the myriad tests and scans needed to figure out what exact kind of lymphoma with which we were dealing.

David was a key driver in what led me to want to change my career, shifting from a TV news journalist to a storyteller of a different kind. I wanted to democratize access for millions of other people out there, to help humanize the experience and understanding of what to do after a cancer diagnosis in the way that David had helped us. That was the genesis of *The Patient Story*, a multi-channel platform with hundreds of in-depth cancer conversations featuring patients, care partners, and top cancer specialists, all with the mission encapsulated by our short tagline: Humanize cancer.

It was through *The Patient Story* that I met Ray Hartjen, a multiple myeloma patient who was diagnosed in 2019. I reached out to Ray via social media after reading about his diagnosis. Since Ray was very public with his treatment, both on social platforms and in the media, I asked if he would share his personal patient story with our *The Patient Story* community.

From the beginning, it was clear that his was a voice that would help so many people out there. Ray was open, honest, and raw in recounting his experience, especially after getting a chronic blood cancer diagnosis of multiple myeloma. His three-part story series clearly resonated with thousands of people seeking to understand that they were and are not alone—his story has hit more than 60,000 views in just over a year.

His commitment has transcended opening up to help others— total strangers. Ray has been actively responding to comments and offering support for those who seek it, especially those newer in their myeloma experience and in their own advocacy journey.

And the passion Ray brings is more important than ever. Cancer stories like Ray's begin as patients undergo testing and arrive at a diagnosis. Unfortunately, more and more patient stories begin each and every day.

Through the compilation of current data on population-based cancer occurrence and outcomes using incidence data collected by central cancer registries and mortality data collected by the National Center for Health Statistics, the American Cancer Society annually estimates the number of new cancer cases in the United States. In 2023, that number is projected to be just under *two million new cancer diagnoses.*

Studies estimate between 30 to 40 percent of Americans will be diagnosed with cancer at some point in their lifetime, with some forecasts even higher. According to the National Cancer Institute (NCI), in the US, men have a one in two chance and women have a one in three chance of being diagnosed with cancer during their lifetimes.[1]

Each diagnosis ignites a journey into a black space filled with uncertainty for patients, their care partners, and their families. Those same questions that plagued me and my family are shared by so many others. But that's the point—as much as it feels like it, none of us is alone. That's the power of sharing our stories. While no two people have the same exact experience, each story has an exponential power to empathize, educate, inspire, and motivate.

Ray's book, *Me, Myself & My Multiple Myeloma*, is the beginning of his personal patient story, and only the beginning, for I'm certain he has much more to experience and share. In telling his story thus far, he serves as a valuable resource for the cancer patient and patient caregiver communities. In the pages that follow, you'll read an unflinching account of multiple myeloma treatment and the impact on body and soul, not just of the patient, but of those of the people around Ray who found themselves having to grapple with and reconcile a cancer diagnosis in their "new normal," as well.

I want to thank Ray for trusting me and our platform to help tell some of his story and for continuing his steadfast and deep dedication to putting pen to paper, serving others in his mission to capture all the lows, super-lows, and some silver linings after his cancer diagnosis to help connect dots for others searching for connection in their cancer experiences.

For you, the reader, who may be a cancer patient and/or a caregiver, I ask you, "What is your story?" I hope you'll consider the power of your voice and experience and share it with our community at *The Patient Story*, which now reaches millions of views monthly.

My story, like Ray's and yours, continues. I'm so grateful to say I am still in remission years later, blessed with a growing family, and celebrate life daily by dedicating it to our wonderfully inspiring community of cancer patients and care partners everywhere.

Stephanie Chuang, founder, The Patient Story community

Chapter 1

D-DAY

My life changed on March 11, 2019. I know that reads a touch overly dramatic, and I know that life is changed every day. But, on that day, my life took a sharp departure from where it had been going.

At least, the direction it had been going in my mind.

March 11, 2019, was my D-Day, my diagnosis day, when, just nineteen days before my fifty-fifth birthday, I was diagnosed with multiple myeloma. At the time, it seemed like everything had changed when I went from a normal guy to a guy now staring down a new normal. And since, I'd like to think the very narrative of my life has changed significantly.

It was a slow trek to a final diagnosis, and in my mind, my story changed over the several weeks leading up to March 11. But, as with most stories, before we get to one point, we have to go back in time to provide a bit of context. So, here it goes.

Twenty-five years ago, my feet and knees began to tell me I needed an exercise regimen that didn't include running, so, like many others,

I got into cycling, at first just plowing around on a mountain bike as a curb jumper to get some exercise, then graduating to road biking, where I put in a couple thousand miles each and every year, including in 2018. Cycling was a big part of my exercise program and, at times, the only part. Riding the bike kept me healthy and fit, and it allowed me to pretty much eat and drink whatever I wanted, and I typically wanted to eat and drink more and more and more.

Cycling was something I couldn't give up—it was a non-negotiable—so I kept at it, even when I developed hemorrhoids, and I continued on even as those hemorrhoids became more problematic. It wasn't a painful condition at all, but the bleeding was disconcerting. So after trying darn near everything, including giving up the bike for two months, I made an appointment with my gastroenterologist in September 2018 as a follow-up to my February colonoscopy, where, in passing, he said rather casually, "Oh, and you do have some hemorrhoids."

At my appointment with his physician's assistant, she stressed that hemorrhoids are relatively normal and won't turn into cancer. So I had that going for me, I guess. She proceeded to ask how much bleeding I was experiencing, and I didn't really know how to answer that. I don't know if it was a lot or a little, but I told her I was of the opinion that blood coming from anywhere, especially, you know, from . . . well, down there . . . was too much blood. I steadfastly refuse to believe I'm alone in that opinion.

Pushing further, she asked if I was hemorrhaging, and I told her I didn't even know what that meant, but it sounded extraordinary, so I guess, no, I wasn't hemorrhaging. But, just in case, she thought it would be a good idea to get a routine blood test and wrote a test requisition.

And that's where my journey really began.

That first blood test showed I was slightly anemic, with my hemoglobin at 11.9, a bit below the low end of the range (the HGB range is generally 11.7–16.7, with the Mayo Clinic advising the normal range for men being 13.5–17.5). It was the first time any high-level blood value of mine had ever been out of range, and the last blood test I had in July 2017 showed no indications of any high-level abnormalities. But, as the HGB count was just a little low, we wanted to confirm the count with another follow-up blood test to see if maybe it was an aberration.

Before I made an appointment for another blood draw to be tested, I had an accident on the bike. On October 7, right at the end of my four-mile warmup and just at the point where I typically crank it up, a flat front tire caused my bike to slide out from under me as I was making a high-speed right turn. As I fell, I thought, "Wow, I'm going down for the first time in about thirty years."

When that thought was going through my head, I was about 45 degrees to the road. The next conscious thought I had, as my eyes opened and I saw a woman kneeling down beside me with her hand on my chest, was *I'm fine.* I actually said it aloud. The woman, who later introduced herself as Suzie, said, "No, you're not. You've been in an accident, you were unconscious, and you're bleeding quite a bit."

Really? Well, okay, then. I guess that explains the group of four to five people gathered around a middle-aged cyclist lying in the middle of the road, which, as I write about it, doesn't seem remotely "fine" at all.

Suzie and another eyewitness said I was unconscious for about five minutes. I'm pretty sure it wasn't that long, as we all tend to exaggerate, right? You know, like when an earthquake rolls past and you swear it lasted for a minute, but when you check the geology site, you see it lasted for seven seconds. If you've ever lived in California, you know what I'm referring to.

I'm not certain I was unconscious for five minutes, but it was long enough to require an ambulance ride to a trauma center and the diagnoses of a severe concussion, three fractures to my orbital bone, and a nifty laceration under my right eyebrow that took a considerable time to suture.

Ah, good times.

So my misadventures on the bike drew my attention away from anemic blood values and follow-up appointments for a handful of weeks. The next thing I knew, it was the holidays and a particularly busy time for me professionally. It was December 7 before I had my blood drawn again for testing.

For whatever reason, I didn't hear back about the results, and, being busy with the holidays, I didn't ask about them until mid-January. That's when we received confirmation about the anemic value from September, as the December draw recorded an HGB value of 11.5, slightly lower still.

Okay, so anemic I was. From there, my medical journey pivoted from determining *if* I was anemic to *why* I was anemic. The effort to determine why began with yet another blood test.

Test three was designed to be a bit more expansive than the previous complete blood counts, or CBCs. Test three was to check for iron, ferrites, and the like, to determine if perhaps I was experiencing internal bleeding. The good news from that February 4 blood test was that those values were all within normal ranges. The bad news was my HGB value had dropped to 10.3. At this point in time, my gastroenterologist referred me to a hematologist.

I had a referral for a name, Dr. Kavitha Raj, but I didn't have a phone number. Looking her up, I saw she was a hematologist/oncologist. An *oncologist,* as in a doctor who diagnoses and treats cancer. I think this was the first time the thought of a possible cancer diagnosis slipped into my mind.

It was clear the seriousness of my anemia had escalated, so I was Johnny on the spot with my follow-up referral. In addition to my consultation with the doctor, my February 14 appointment featured a number of blood vials drawn for a deep dive into what might be ailing me. Unsurprisingly, my anemia was again confirmed, this time with an HGB value of 11.2. But that HGB score was the least of my worries.

More problematic was the level of protein markers in my blood. Until then, my anemia could have been explained away as a result of somewhat "lazy" bone marrow not producing enough red blood cells. The protein markers suggested something different—and a lot more problematic. That's when my wife, Lori, and I first heard the words "lymphoma" and "multiple myeloma."

We didn't have a definitive diagnosis yet, and there were still other potential root causes, but in my head, I was beginning to accept that my particular diagnosis was likely going to be something ending in an *A,* and something somewhat sinister at that.

The long diagnosis period was playing itself out, slowly uncovering the root cause of my anemia.

Going over my blood test results and pointing out the protein markers, Dr. Raj shared with us that two very real possibilities were lymphoma or multiple myeloma. But, in learning more about the two diseases, between the two, it was a case of "careful what you wish for."

Lymphoma is a curable disease. Multiple myeloma is incurable yet treatable, and Dr. Raj added that "many people live a long, long time."

So . . . great. Two relatively poor choices. One disease is curable but perhaps more deadly in the short term. The other disease is less deadly in the short-term but a chronic condition and incurable.

Which, of course, left me wondering if there was a third choice. "What's behind that third curtain, Monty?" Unfortunately, as so many have discovered, health care isn't a game of *Let's Make a Deal.*

Close to a final diagnosis, the protein markers pushed Dr. Raj to order two additional tests to hopefully get to a definitive cause: a PET scan and a bone marrow biopsy. The PET scan was to get a picture of what might be going on in my body, and relative to a lot of medical tests, a PET scan is almost a joy to experience. Compared to a bone marrow biopsy, a PET scan is like Christmas morning, on a beach, holding a winning super lotto ticket in your hand.

Here's a pro tip, from me to you: a bone marrow biopsy should not be considered recreationally. It's not a hobby.

When Dr. Raj first broached a bone marrow biopsy, I responded with a little smirk and a cough-like, nervous chuckle. She looked at me, almost defensively, even somewhat confused, and said, "What?"

I replied, "Come on, Doc. A bone marrow biopsy is preceded by its reputation, and it's not exactly a good one at that."

Dr. Raj said something along the lines of, "Some patients feel fifteen to thirty seconds of pressure or discomfort." And, she added, some patients don't really feel much of anything at all.

Ha. That memory actually makes me laugh as I type. Even as she spoke, I knew better, of course.

On biopsy day, the physician's assistant, the one who was going to perform the test, had a different spiel. As she closed the door to the exam room, she said, "You're going to feel discomfort like you've never felt before."

Cutting to the chase, let me say that her description—in my particular case, at least—was a bit more accurate.

I'd show a picture of the needle she used to insert into my bone to acquire my bone marrow samples, but I can't bring myself to do so. I have more bone marrow biopsies in my future, and I'd just as soon know as little about this little test of horrors (okay, granted, perhaps a bit dramatic) as I can.

Lori was, and continues to be, by my side through all of my doctor visits, and I'm extremely grateful, for the journey to a cancer diagnosis can be daunting and exhausting, both mentally and physically. But I wish she hadn't been in the exam room for the biopsy. It's not easy seeing a loved one in that much discomfort, and I know I didn't enjoy seeing Lori engulfed in the discomfort of childbirth. Likewise, she didn't enjoy seeing what I was going through—so much so, she had to leave the room. She described herself as "traumatized" for at least a month afterward.

All the tests prior to the bone marrow biopsy were directional, guiding us to a diagnosis through a process of elimination. They provided indicators of what might be the cause, but they were not definitive. You can infer a great deal of probability, but the only way to really know what's going on is to get inside where it's going on and take a look. In my case, that was inside my bones, at the bone marrow.

When the lab looked at my bone marrow, it became clear: an aggressive form of multiple myeloma had taken over 90 percent of my bone marrow. Somehow, six months after having a consultation about hemorrhoids, of all things, I now had a diagnosis of multiple myeloma, a blood cancer.

I was extremely fortunate to discover my multiple myeloma in the manner in which I did. Often, patients are diagnosed after suffering fractures from weakened bones, often at advanced levels of the disease. A great many patients suffer compression fractures of the spine and in determining a root cause, are diagnosed with multiple myeloma.

In time, I met a fellow patient in a group session who shared his story. He went to bed one night measuring five feet, nine inches tall. In the morning, when he got out of bed and took his first step, he suffered multiple compression fractures in his spine. From those steps forward to today, he now stands five feet, six inches tall.

As I wrote, I consider myself fortunate. This disease was well established in my body, and it would have eventually been discovered.

Discovering it before I was too symptomatic allowed me to take pro-active action, actions that continue to this day.

Oh, and to close the loop, my hemorrhoids are no longer as prob-lematic. So I have that going for me. Which, evoking Bill Murray's character, Carl, in the movie *Caddyshack*, is nice.

I've mentioned that multiple myeloma is an incurable blood cancer, but I haven't shared much about it. Multiple myeloma—also known as Kahler's disease, although I never knew that until I looked it up—is a cancer of plasma cells, a type of white blood cell in the human bone marrow.

Multiple myeloma fools the body into thinking cancerous cells are normal plasma cells, and the cancer thus multiplies, relatively unchecked. In time, if left untreated, multiple myeloma attacks the bones, immune system, kidneys, and, as mentioned along my diagnosis journey, red blood cell counts.

Multiple myeloma is a relatively rare cancer, although not quite as rare as to my liking, as I wouldn't have minded one bit if it had skipped over me. Anyway, less than 200,000 cases of multiple myeloma are diagnosed each year.

The causes of multiple myeloma are unclear. However, there is a close correlation between multiple myeloma and a condition called monoclonal gammopathy of unknown significance, or MGUS, where there is an excess of protein molecules, called immunoglobulins, in a patient's blood.

My medical team suggested that somewhere along the line I experienced a genetic mutation that my body didn't self-correct. Then it became "normal" for my body to have myeloma cells lying about, free to replicate and grow unabated.

There is no cure for multiple myeloma at this time, but it is treatable. The Multiple Myeloma Research Foundation (MMRF) states that multiple myeloma can be a highly manageable disease.

I had never heard of multiple myeloma before I began my fight with it. And, despite the prevalence of information online, I haven't dug too much into the particulars. I understand the average life expectancy after diagnosis is five years, but I don't want to hear anything about that. I want to be in this fight for a heck of a lot longer than that.

Some patients and patient caregivers flock to the readiness of information on the internet. Shoot, Lori practically has an MD degree from Google University. For me, I don't want to know step 100 in my fight. Rather, I want to know about step one. Let me take care of that one first. I figure I'll deal with number two when the time comes.

Chapter 2

SAY IT AIN'T SO

Okay, so I have multiple myeloma, an incurable but treatable blood cancer. That was the "so what?" Next came the "now what?"

Perhaps nothing is as private to individuals as their health. Sharing information about your health is a personal decision, and as such, there's no right or wrong.

My diagnosis was already shared the moment it came out. After all, Lori was sitting there alongside me during every appointment leading up to the diagnosis. What I heard, she heard, and that allowed me to sidestep one undoubtedly difficult conversation, that being informing my spouse of my diagnosis.

During my diagnostic appointments, Lori was strong, as solid as a rock. However, at that last appointment, or maybe it was the appointment before, it all caught up with her as we were leaving the building. In the car, she broke down and sobbed. A serious and chronic disease—a disease like cancer—can be a heavy, emotional load to carry for both patient and loved ones alike.

I patted her hand as I was driving and told her not to worry. I told her I was going to be around to grow old with her.

Lori and I haven't really talked about my—or our—mortality. Years later, as I began writing this manuscript and the topic of a book came up, she started to share. She recounted the days after my—and very much *our*—diagnosis, and she recalled being momentarily lost in the thoughts of "What am I going to do without him?" In just a couple of spoken sentences, she was choking up. The emotional weight of the topic, even over three years after my initial diagnosis, led us to quickly and awkwardly change the topic.

It's still too much to bear for both of us, even after all we've been through.

I remember reading an account years ago of a cancer patient who didn't share his diagnosis with anyone, including his wife and family. It was his secret, literally, all the way through his treatment, a marked decline in his health, and his eventual death. The article quoted his family as speculating that he kept it a secret to not burden them. Interestingly, his family was a bit bent out of shape by that decision. They wanted to be with him. They wanted to go through the journey with him, supporting and caring as they could. He might not have needed it, but they felt as though *they* needed it. They wanted it.

It's an interesting point of view that I would be reminded of repeatedly as I began and continued my fight with cancer.

That cancer patient wasn't right or wrong. He just was. I've met others much like him. There's a patient in my support group who has told practically no one about his diagnosis. His immediate family knows, but they're sworn to secrecy. His own mother doesn't know. I'd place his age at late-fifties, early-sixties, making his mother approximately eighty. I assume he just doesn't want to burden his elderly mother with any additional—and in his mind, unnecessary—worry.

Another patient in the group has only told his mother, and the only reason he did was because he lives with her and there would be no hiding the fact after a couple of required surgeries. Other than that, no one knows of his pancreatic cancer and treatment other than his medical team and the members of our support group.

Their decisions.

For me, Lori already knew, and I felt as though I needed to get the word out. However, in doing so, I quickly discovered telling others wasn't particularly easy.

I mean, it's easy to just blurt out something. But emotionally, I found it to be very difficult to inform those close to me—family, friends, co-workers, and others in my personal and professional communities.

As with a lot of endeavors, getting started was the hardest part.

I don't mean making the decision to publicly share a diagnosis. For me, that decision came easily. It was actually conducting the first conversation. I wish I had thought it out a bit better. Unfortunately, there is no how-to guide, or at least it didn't occur to me to search for one. But maybe I should have practiced in front of a mirror or something.

I decided to let others know, and I felt I couldn't waste much time in doing so as I was certain that the news would spread through the grapevine quickly. It was important for me to deliver the news personally and factually, and to assuage any fears and let people know I was okay.

I even cooked up what I thought was a sound strategy. I'd start with family first, and I'd work my way from east to west to make sure time zones wouldn't postpone my difficult conversations to another day. That way, I'd avoid any unnecessary delays that might open windows for back-channel family conversations that would spill the beans for those unaware. They'd all hear it from me, and that was important to me.

My first call was to my daughter Olivia, who was halfway through the second semester of her first year at Vanderbilt Law School. In hindsight, I probably should have just picked up Lori's phone and Facetimed her, bringing up my diagnosis during our conversation. After all, Facetime conversations between those two aren't that uncommon. Unfortunately, I wasn't that clever.

Instead, I texted her, telling her I needed to speak with her. That, of course, set her alarms off. I mean, with text messaging and email, Olivia and I don't actually speak to each other very often. In fact, someone her age, twenty-three at the time, might not even know they can talk on that mobile, handheld, Instagram-surfing machine of theirs.

In her mind, something had to be wrong, and when she called back, she was already on the verge of tears. It didn't take long before we were both crying as I struggled to tell my baby girl about my diagnosis. It was not easy—by far, the worst, most difficult conversation I've ever had on the phone.

Then my crisis communication learning curve ramped up. My parents in Kansas were next, and it was only a tad bit easier. Fewer tears. At least, I think so. Next up, my son Raymond, at school in Santa Clara. And that was a bit better still. Then I circled back across the country to my sister Ruth in Cincinnati, where the tears came again when talking about being an uncle to her relatively young children.

Just when I thought I had my act together, our friends Paul and Donna Truex pulled a drop by to talk in person about a trip we were planning together for September of that year—a month in Europe, starting with the Italian Grand Prix at Monza and ending with Oktoberfest in Munich. I walked them into the kitchen, where Lori then joined us, immediately blurting out, "So did you tell them?"

Donna and Paul eyeballed one another, then glanced back at us, clearly wondering what they were about to be told.

Yeah, no escaping explaining that introduction. Thus, the next step in my learning curve was conducting face-to-face, in-person conversations. Again, not easy. But something that, with practice, became a lot more matter-of-fact. By the weekend, I had shared my news a number of times, and then I inadvertently outed myself to a much broader audience online.

During a sloppy band rehearsal in my kitchen, my first prescription of Revlimid, one of my prescribed immunotherapy drugs, was delivered to my house. My Chronic Padres bandmate Scott Sorochak filmed a quick little video that I shared with my family. Then, for whatever reason, I thought I'd tweet out to Lance Armstrong and the Livestrong Foundation that I had started kicking cancer's butt. After all, no one reads my X feed—of that I was fairly certain.

Turns out some people in my professional network saw the tweet (what a post was called back then)—a lot of them actually, with thirteen of them "liking" the tweet and some sending me messages of encouragement, one via text message on my phone. Oddly, Lance and Livestrong didn't reply. I don't know if my intended audience ever saw the tweet among the heavy stream I'm sure they get daily. But a little chunk of my followers did for sure.

I shared my diagnosis because I wanted people to know about it from me. I wanted to make it personal, and I didn't want friends and colleagues to hear about it from others. In hindsight, that was a bit naive. I literally have thousands of contacts in my personal and professional networks; some, of course, I know better than others. Still, having a full-time job and a host of other responsibilities, I didn't have time to spend ten minutes personally with everyone. Short of big Facebook and LinkedIn posts, which aren't personal at all, the majority of the people in my circles would find out over time, likely from others.

I decided to share my multiple myeloma diagnosis because I wanted people to know. But that, too, was probably too simplistic. It's a conversation that has cropped up in my support group on many occasions.

Sharing a diagnosis of a medical condition can be surprisingly complicated. Initially, I thought of it strictly as a one-way dialogue, with me informing and others listening and learning. Of course, that's simply not how the vast majority of human interactions work. There's going to be a reaction, a response from others. Before sharing their diagnoses, patients should think about their desired outcomes from those conversations and level set their expectations.

The first cancer patients I got to know in my long-sheltered life were those in my support group, which I started attending within a couple of weeks of my final diagnosis. In talking with them about sharing diagnoses and treatment updates, a great many of them expressed frustration with others. Their annoyance sprung from receiving platitudes like, "You're going to be alright," "You got this," and similar. And, as the days, months, and years go by, it becomes a recurring frustration for many of them. So much so, they keep quiet about their health and medical treatment around others, keeping their thoughts and feelings bottled up inside, rarely letting them bubble up, and in many cases, only letting them bubble up and out during group.

What those patients want is for their friends and family to acknowledge the fact that there are days they feel like crap, days when they're scared, days they just want to lie in bed and try to get over their treatments. They want empathy, not cheerleading.

Personally, I prefer cheerleading. I think I'm my biggest cheerleader, and for years, I've firmly believed people can manifest a great deal of their destiny through the power of positive thought.

Group, however, continues to teach me that while we as humans have so much more in common than we do in differences, the differences quite often have a significantly larger and more profound impact. In group, I've discovered a surprisingly large number of cancer patients get discouraged about their network of friends, with more than one stating something like, "You find out who your real friends are."

Now, I don't know the particular circumstances of what's brought them to that conclusion. I know I don't feel that way, and I will forever try my hardest to never allow myself to think that way. In group, I've jumped to their friends' defense, suggesting they should consider cutting them a bit of a break. And here's why.

Let me speak for myself, only. Over the years, I have refused to acknowledge the pregnancy of a woman until she first tells me she is pregnant. She could be in labor, pushing her baby's crowning head out, and I wouldn't say a thing about being pregnant. Why? Well, I've stood right next to a woman who was not pregnant when another person asked her, "So when are you expecting?"

Totally awkward. And potentially awkward situations like that created a deep-set fear within me—I never want to open my mouth and place myself in that sort of situation. It drove my emotional intelligence—my emotional quotient, or EQ, if you will—to precariously low levels. Handicapped as I was, and self-imposed at that, I typically don't speak of pregnancies. Ever.

I used the same principle with significant others. I had more or less stopped asking about significant others in 1993, when I asked a graduate school classmate of mine where her husband was. When she replied with a sneer, "Not here," I pretty much decided it was better to be safe than sorry, so if I wasn't absolutely, positively certain a couple was still together, I'd hold my tongue about inquiring about a friend's significant other until something came up in conversation where I knew the coast was clear.

I didn't have the emotional intelligence to deal with personal, emotional, and even marginally difficult conversations. And I don't think I'm alone in being in a space like that.

It's a pity. I'm certain I've missed out on a lot in my past simply because I avoided meaningful, human-to-human conversations. I've particularly missed out on sharing with others that I care about them and what was happening in their lives, all because I wanted to avoid a potentially awkward moment, even if there was a low probability that moment would ever occur.

And then there is an example of an experience that hit much closer to home, one that I shared with my group. In May 2019, just a couple of months after my diagnosis, the oncology center where we all go for treatment had a cancer open house, about a six-hour day with exercises, speakers, and even crafts. About twenty-five cancer patients were in attendance, and at one point in the afternoon, several employees of the center came into the room to celebrate with us the upcoming retirement of one of the facilitators.

During that time, one of the center's team members spoke to the group, sharing how much she'd enjoyed working with them and noti-fying us all that that day was going to be her last day at the center, as she would be going out on medical leave. One of my fellow patients said, "Good luck, and I look forward to you coming back to work." The employee, choking back tears in what was obviously an emotional moment for her, replied, "I won't be coming back. It's a permanent leave; I've been diagnosed with ALS."

Lou Gehrig's disease.

At that moment, all the air went out of the room, and a full room of cancer patients sat stunned, silent, and in disbelief. No one said anything.

At all.

Not one person got up and hugged her.

No one did anything but sit in stunned silence.

I had never met her before. I didn't—and still don't—know her. I frequently think back on that moment with regret, and even a bit of shame. I so wish I had said something. But like everyone else, including some of the people I had heard previously say, "You find out who your real friends are," I didn't say anything.

Why?

Because we all, every single one of us, didn't know what to say. That singular moment was too big for us. The thing is, as cancer patients, we all *knew better*! A great many of us had expressed strong, negative feelings about expecting better from others when sharing our diagnoses. Yet, in the moment of need from another, we collectively—and me, individually—failed.

As I wrote above, sharing information about a diagnosis or treatment can be complex and extraordinarily difficult. So here's an idea for patients, caregivers, friends, and co-workers alike: How about we give each other a break from judgment?

I totally get why some people don't reach out to me to talk about my cancer and how I'm doing. It's the same reason I've been afraid to talk about pregnancies or significant others and the same reason I haven't reached out to friends in the past. When I haven't spoken to someone in a decade or more, I think to myself, *What am I going to say?* Likewise, when a friend is going through a tough time, what am I going to say?

When I hear someone has been diagnosed with ALS, cancer, or some other serious health condition, what am I going to say?

I think I know now, and it's really pretty simple. I'll just fess up and say, "I don't know what to say. But I love you. I care about you. And I want to be there for you. I'm hoping you and I can push through this together and figure it all out. Just know that I'm with you."

As the saying goes, you live, you learn.

These days, I ask women how their pregnancies are going. I inquire about the well-being of significant others. And I listen. If I find myself in an awkward conversation, so be it—it will not be so bad that I can't work my way out of it.

The best relationships are the relationships that dive deeper, that go below the superficial. They press us to understand emotions better, both ours and theirs. It's a lesson I continue to learn, and it's undoubtedly improving my relationships, making them more meaningful.

It's a shame it took so long.

Chapter 3

GETTING INTO THE FIGHT

Getting to a final diagnosis of multiple myeloma took some time, and it was time that weighed heavily on me. I had plenty to think about, and after a short while, it was, "What am I going to do about this?"

I've always been proactive and accountable. I'd rather be doing than being done upon, and as I was beginning to feel a bit helpless, I sought an opportunity to take back a degree of control.

The journey to diagnosis felt like jumping through a lot of hoops. Many doctors' appointments, many needles drawing blood, many appointments for scans and biopsies. Cancer was dictating my days and my weeks, and that was taking its toll on me mentally.

I wasn't in charge; I wasn't the boss. Cancer was moving into the corner office, becoming the boss.

That wasn't going to cut it.

While waiting for that final diagnosis, I decided my first steps to taking back some control, to being proactively accountable for my response to what ailed me, was my diet—the nutrients I put into my body. From years before, I remembered a radio interview I had heard with Patrick Quillin, author of *Beating Cancer with Nutrition*, so I searched for the book and added it to my cart. And, before check-out, our good friends at Amazon suggested I take a look at *The Cancer-Fighting Kitchen*, written by Rebecca Katz, which I also put into my cart and purchased.

My diet was already pretty good and fairly well-balanced. Red meat wasn't often included in our meals, and, in fact, a great many of our meals were vegetarian, thanks to the preferences of our son, Raymond. I may have over-indulged in candy from time to time, a side effect of Lori always having M&Ms and the like around the house, but it was never too problematic because long, fast rides on the bike kept the weight off.

One thing that certainly needed to change, though, was my alcohol consumption. In speaking with my doctor during the run-up to a diagnosis, when she asked about alcohol, I estimated between seven and ten drinks a week. Lori, by nature, is quick to defend her loved ones, and she piped in about how I have a glass of wine with dinner or after dinner most every night, and the doctor kind of nodded.

But not so fast. Yes, sure, a glass of wine a night equals seven drinks a week. But then there's band practice, which often included a drink or two, and meeting up with buddies for a beer or two, and social occasions where there would be—any guesses?—a drink or two. Then, there was the occasional bender, a music festival, or an afternoon at a football game, and, well, it wouldn't take a Newtonian brain for mathematics to calculate an average number of weekly drinks for me to have been . . . well, let's be a bit charitable and say, "A touch above seven to ten" a week.

I know what you're thinking, and you're right. My doctor also thought cutting back from that baseline level would be a good idea.

Cancer has a lot of similarities to other cells, and one is they love—crave—sugar. It's quick and easy fuel. The sugar buzz a child gets on Halloween is just the cumulation of a whole bunch of cells being jacked up on sugar.

Most of the alcohol I drank didn't contain any added sugar and didn't have a very high sugar content. But, from a caloric standpoint, they contained empty calories, nothing that really helped me function, much less fight off a disease. Plus, alcohol placed a burden on my liver, the filter for my blood.

For me, the decision to cut back on my intake of alcohol was easy. What was much more difficult was actually cutting back on it. After all, I do love a glass of wine or a tumbler of bourbon. But, these days, I drink a lot less, and I'm convinced my body is better off for it.

Some cancer patients have a "journey" with cancer. Others have a "fight" with cancer. I believe it's more than just simple semantics. It comes down to a patient's personality and how he or she views things, including, very much, spirituality.

Fight or journey, it's not a reflection of the combative nature of a patient. Anyone who has ever sat in a chemotherapy infusion or a radiation treatment chair is one heck of a combative individual.

Lots of cancer pundits, including a great many doctors, perhaps even a majority of doctors, disagree with me on the journey versus the fight idea. They'll state that treating cancer is about living with cancer, a journey. A fight or a battle carries the connotation of war, and with it, a clear winner or loser. Many of us know patients who have lost their lives to cancer. In no way should they be considered losers.

The idea of fighting cancer goes back a long way, but it really gained momentum over fifty years ago when US President Richard Nixon declared a "war on cancer" when he signed the National Cancer Act of 1971. The war metaphor was required at the time, increasing much-needed research funding and cancer activism. Cancer research is Expensive, with an uppercase *E*, and there's nothing like wartime propaganda to literally rally the troops.

For me, I prefer to look at my treatment for multiple myeloma as a fight. Simply, I'm more motivated and inspired by fighting analogies and metaphors.

When I think about a journey, I think about one of those long road trips of my childhood, in our car, pounding down seemingly endless miles of sun-soaked interstate highway. The only companionship was family—my parents and sister. Even alongside family, those long trips in the backseats of Cadillacs and Lincolns were interminable. The joy certainly wasn't in the journey, but much more so once we reached the destination.

I'm surely not going to cozy up to multiple myeloma for a journey to some as-of-yet undefined destination. No, sir.

I'm going to meet multiple myeloma in the middle of the ring, and we're going to battle it out. Each test thus far has gotten me more and more battle-tested. The fight analogy gets me fired up for the next round.

So to each patient their own; while some have journeys, I have a fight.

The concept of fighting cancer with nutrition is perhaps best compared to gardening. A gardener wants to prepare their soil to nourish, accommodate, and promote the growth and health of the plants they want to grow (healthy cells for the cancer fighter) while, at the same time, making the soil inhospitable to the weeds (cancer cells) they want to kill off and prevent from coming back.

Getting to my final diagnosis, I decided it was time for me to clean up my diet and get to tending to my garden. First up, that alcohol thing. Some types of alcohol are better, nutritionally, than others. But make no mistake about it, no type of alcohol is a good nutrient for your body.

Regardless, I wasn't going to give up alcohol entirely. Rather shamefully, I like it too much. No, I'm talking about being drunk. Although, I can't lie to you and tell you I haven't had some extraordinarily fun time under the influence of alcohol. I wasn't going to give up alcohol completely because I like having the occasional drink too much. However, seven to ten drinks—or a touch *above* seven to ten drinks—a week immediately fell down to one or two drinks a week.

It wasn't particularly easy. I used to enjoy a glass of bourbon two or three days a week. In the first six months of my treatment, I had just a single glass, a birthday gift to myself.

Oh, and those handfuls of M&Ms were wiped out completely. I tried my best to break up with processed sugar. While sugar had never been my best friend, it certainly wasn't public enemy number one for me, either. It's still not. But it's on my ten most wanted list. Or perhaps, my ten least wanted list.

Of course, good nutrition isn't just cutting down on alcohol and sugar, although that's a good start for darn near anyone. I also bumped up the amount of fruits and vegetables and added fish, whole grains, and legumes as regular components of my weekly diet. I continued with lean proteins like chicken breast. Also, I began shopping organic for the first time ever.

I had always avoided organic food because of the cost premium. Now, however, organic foods, particularly vegetables, have become a priority. In my mind, the concept was simple and logical: if my body was already struggling with abnormal cells, why would I want to put additional chemicals in there, some of them cancer-causing and cancer-promoting carcinogens? Same with cooking methods, like smoking fatty meats.

The two books I ordered have been insightful and valuable, particularly *The Cancer-Fighting Kitchen*. First, the recipes produce some tasty vittles, and that's important. What I really like about the book, though, and the reason I promote it every chance I get, is the various ways it is organized to assist the cancer patient and their caregiver(s).

The Cancer-Fighting Kitchen has a section dealing with symptoms and recommendations. If the reader is feeling nauseated or fatigued or suffering from side effects like diarrhea or constipation, the author suggests certain recipes. There's a section on treatments and recipe suggestions for the days preceding and following treatments, as well as recommendations for the day(s) of treatment. There's even a quick guide for improving the taste of food if a patient is suffering from side effects of treatment that affect taste—for example, everything tasting metallic.

I'm far from an expert in cancer-fighting nutrition, but a seemingly great place to start is a Mediterranean diet, with meals built around plant-based foods—vegetables, fruits, herbs, nuts, beans, and whole grains—and moderate amounts of dairy, poultry, and eggs. Lots of fish, but not so much red meat.

Changing my diet gave me a sense of being proactive, of taking steps to seize back control from cancer and to show cancer who's boss in this particular arena. Importantly, improving upon my diet was a boost to my morale. Sure, I spend a lot of time preparing food, eating, and cleaning up, as I eat smaller "micro" meals and snacks almost all day long, but that's okay because at least I'm in the fight.

Does reading about food make you hungry? I know writing about it makes me hungry. So let me share with you one of my favorite recipes from *The Cancer-Fighting Kitchen*, a quick-and-easy snack or appetizer.

Cannellini Bean Dip with Kalamata Olives[2]

- 2 cups cooked cannellini beans or 1 15-ounce can, drained, rinsed, and mixed with a spritz of fresh lemon juice and a pinch of salt
- ½ teaspoon minced garlic
- 3 tablespoons extra-virgin olive oil
- 2 tablespoons water
- 2 tablespoons freshly squeezed lemon juice
- ½ teaspoon sea salt
- Pinch of cayenne
- ¼ cup pitted Kalamata olives, rinsed
- ¼ cup chopped fresh basil
- Combine all the ingredients in a food processor and process until smooth.[2]

Slice fresh, organic vegetables and use this as a dip, or use it as a spread on bread. I like to use it on my bagel in the morning, topped off with avocado. Give it a try—I think you'll like it!

Chapter 4

A PROCESS, NOT AN EVENT

I mmediately upon my myeloma diagnosis, I started treatment. I also had yet another test to go through.

As multiple myeloma manifests itself in bone marrow, over time, it can seep into bones and weaken them. Unexpected, unexplained bone fractures are often the first notable symptom in many patients.

I went through a PET (positron emission tomography) scan to determine if there were any hot spots in my skeletal system. It's a simple procedure for the patient, but yet another one that comes with a bit of a mental hurdle. You see, for a PET scan, the patient is injected with a radioactive tracer drug, and the metabolic activity in the body is then picked up by the imaging.

Patients will actually give off low-grade radiation for up to six hours after the procedure. So much so, patients should not be around pregnant women during that time period.

I mean, it's a little spooky, right?

So I willingly received an injection of a radioactive isotope directly into my vascular system, and I did it with a bit of a shrug. First, I knew Lori wasn't pregnant; second, I knew that much worse would be pumped into me as my treatment progressed.

Fortunately, my PET scan results came back negative. There were a couple of what Dr. Raj described as "cloudy" spots in the images, but nothing that would require me to go through a sequence of radiation treatments. I had dodged that bullet by getting diagnosed relatively early. Despite 90 percent of my bone marrow being cancerous, the disease had not made too much progress into my bones.

One of my new friends in my support group had not been so fortunate with his myeloma diagnosis. On top of the standard induction treatment, he endured a great many trips for radiation, which comes with its own laundry list of unpleasant side effects.

Radiation treatments are designed to kill cancer cells, or at least slow their growth. However, there is always collateral damage, with the radiation adversely affecting normal cells within the body. In addition to damaging and killing normal cells, radiation treatments typically come with numerous side effects, including diarrhea, chronic fatigue, nausea and vomiting, urinary and bladder complications, skin problems, and even hair loss.

By avoiding any radiation treatments, my induction treatment for my multiple myeloma consisted of the standard, rather cut-and-dried "RVD" treatment. *R* is for Revlimid, or lenalidomide, a once-a-day tablet I initially took in a cycle of three weeks on, one week off. My induction therapy dose of Revlimid was pretty heavy, 25 mg tablets, as I recall. The *V* is for Velcade, or bortezomib, a once-weekly targeted proteasome inhibitor chemotherapy injection given in the abdomen. The *D* is for Dexamethasone, a steroid taken once a week in a pretty hefty dose—for me, 40 mg once a week.

Then, because of all the potential side effects, and there is a whole host of potential side effects, there were a bunch of other drugs prescribed to keep me healthy, ready, and able to ingest the real cancer-fighters. One was the antiviral acyclovir, a 400 mg tablet taken once a day to ward off shingles. I also took 325 mg of aspirin daily to prevent blood clots.

Like other patients, my induction treatment was prescribed to start immediately, with the expectation of running it for three to six months, leading up to the next likely stage of treatment, a stem cell transplant.

With an initial treatment plan in place, I was finally in the fight! It's exactly where I wanted to be and what I wanted to do.

When Lori and I had met with Dr. Raj to discover the final diagnosis, I had opened the conversation with a simple ask: "Tell me what I have so I can get fighting. Right now, I feel I've been slapped around by cancer—poked and prodded, with a bone marrow biopsy—and I'm ready to get in the fight and throw some punches of my own."

When I started treatment within days of my diagnosis, I felt I was fighting back, and it felt good. Treatment gave me something to take control of, and I embraced it and focused on what I thought I could control—my diet, my physical activity, my medications, and my mental attitude.

I compartmentalized, dealing with the tasks and opportunities immediately in front of me and working on solving for those first. I'd solve for a stem cell transplant when the time came. I took my medicine, literally, and set off to fight my myeloma.

Almost immediately, I suffered through side effects. Digestive issues hit me, but the worst was probably my skin. The high dose of Revlimid caused skin rashes across my chest, neck, and upper arms. And the injection sites for my weekly Velcade shots would leave long swaths of damaged, hardened, bruised, and scarred skin, about four inches long and two inches wide.

The physical side effects of beginning treatment after diagnosis were only the beginning and just part of the story. There was an entire mental and emotional aspect as well.

I don't know what it's like for other patients, but for me, after diagnosis, it was difficult to think about much other than cancer. I suspect it's similar to what other patients experience.

Cancer was pretty much the first thing I thought about upon waking in the morning and the last thing I thought about at night as I fell asleep. And, of course, during the day, the thought was never far from my mind.

I've always had a bit of a "ten-minute rule" throughout my life. I'm not one to dwell on things for too long, to beat myself up about something. The ten-minute rule allows one to react to something—whatever that reaction might be, including throwing a nice pity party—for ten minutes, then move on with some type of positive response. Response versus reaction; I believe there's a difference, and it's not just a different word meaning the same thing.

Anyway, going into that final diagnosis appointment, I told Lori, "Okay, whatever it is, we have the ten-minute rule and then we get on with it."

That turned out to be a bit naive. Try as I might, the ten minutes turned out to be ten (or maybe even more) minutes per hour, every hour, for a couple of weeks! It was a lot of thinking, a lot of realization and acceptance, and the mental aspect of my diagnosis led directly to a steady stream of emotions, which seemed to be cumulative. It was a growing tower of mental and emotional strain.

Almost everything I've done, every challenge I've ever faced, has led up to and ended with some sort of capstone event. Be it academically, professionally, athletically, musically, or whatever, the challenge has been a process—studying, preparing, training, rehearsing, etc.—that ends with an event: a final exam, a deadline, a game, a gig, etc.

Capstone events have always allowed me to build up to a crescendo, peak at the right moment, deliver the goods, then sit back, relax, and plan out the next process for the next big thing to come up.

When I was a kid, Bjorn Borg dominated the Wimbledon tennis tournament, winning five consecutive titles between 1976 and 1980 (not to mention his six career French Open titles, as well). As a boy, I read an article in *Sports Illustrated* titled, "The Beard Has Begun," where the writer chronicled Borg's preparation for the 1981 Wimbledon tournament. Borg always wore a scruffy beard for the two-week tournament, and the article referenced Borg's singular focus on the tournament, so much so that he wouldn't shave. Each look in the mirror and every touch of his face would remind him of his singular priority—preparing for and working his way through the tournament.

Despite being seventeen, I didn't have the need to shave when I read the article, but it did resonate with me, so much so that I can easily find the article in a Google search because its title has been permanently etched in my memory. For decades now, I've let the beard begin as I've worked toward big things—a project at work, a big athletic competition, or something else.

My cancer beard started on March 11. It was symbolic for me in a couple of ways. First, it marked my fight against multiple myeloma, a need to teach those cancer cells a lesson. Cancer may have forced me into this game, but the game was on my home court, and we were going to play by my neighborhood's rules.

Second, I understood from my doctor that any subsequent stem cell transplant would begin with a pretty heavy dose of chemotherapy—several doses, actually—that would likely result in the loss of my hair. So my thought was to grow out my hair and beard and then give it all a ceremonial shave down ahead of the chemotherapy and transplant. Again, it's another game, but I was going to make it my own, doing it my way, with my rules.

On a side note, I can tell you that after four months of growing a beard, I had second thoughts about the entire thing. Shaggy couldn't begin to describe it. And the patchwork of gray was an entirely different matter. I thought about dying it, but I was shocked at how much beard dye costs.

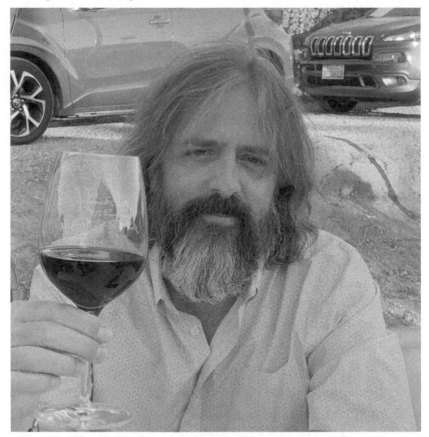

The author sporting the full power of the beard during the summer of 2019.
(Photo courtesy of Lori Hartjen)

Anyway, back on topic.

There I was, with a beard and a relentless, everyday focus on controlling what I could, eating well, exercising, and taking my meds. I was taking the fight to cancer, and my body responded immediately with my HGB rising to 11.8 after one week, then 12.3 after two weeks.

However, unbeknownst to me, my traditional approach to challenges was taking its toll. I was taking an approach that had worked well for leading up and preparing for a capstone moment in time—again, a game or a race, a gig, a big deliverable at work, and the like. Multiple myeloma was different.

After a couple of weeks of complete focus on my fight at hand and a steady escalation of build-up, I experienced a pretty "blue" day. It was a Friday, the end of a work week, and Lori, Raymond, and I were going out for dinner. I was beat, and feeling beat brought on that blue streak.

I was exhausted. It was a cumulative effect of all that mental, emotional, and spiritual strain, and combined, it impacted me physically too. I was flat-out tired, in every single aspect. And I was, in large part, to blame for the self-inflicted wound.

Multiple myeloma is a chronic condition. There's no cure. There's treatment and perhaps, in time, a cure, but right now, it's incurable. In the fight against multiple myeloma, there is no singular capstone moment, no game day or fight night.

My approach to my fight had been built around a faulty model, and I needed to make adjustments. At the end of those first two weeks, I learned there is no one fight night with multiple myeloma. Rather, every night is fight night. Multiple myeloma doesn't lend itself to a training camp-type of mentality, preparing for a big day, a big capstone event, a finish line. Instead, every day is the same fight. It's not about peaking for a day. It's about bringing your best each day. It's not a project; it's a process, a lifestyle—it's life.

Fighting cancer would be something I wake up to every day. With a new dawn comes another game day, a continuation of the contest from the day before, the week before, the month and years before. A new day and a new opportunity to live, and in the process, to show cancer who's boss.

I had learned a lesson, and it was a lesson I could only learn from and by myself, through trial and error. I had to redefine fight night and game day in my mind. Cancer treatment, for me, a patient with a chronic disease, was not ever going to be an event. It was—and continues to be—a process.

In addition to my diet, I continued to exercise as I started my fight with cancer. Exercise has always made me feel good about myself, and while staring down a cancer diagnosis, I needed something to feel good about.

I was still hesitant about getting back to my bicycle after my October 2018 accident. Plus, late winter/early spring rides are a bit chilly, taking some of the fun away from the ride. Anyway, I wasn't too concerned about my cardiovascular fitness. All those years on the bike pounding away the miles had left a lot of deposits in my cardiovascular health bank. I figured now was the time to take out some withdrawals.

Every trip to the doctor I got—and still get—my vital signs taken, including blood pressure and pulse. My pulse is in the mid- to low-fifties, and that's not a resting pulse rate taken when I wake up. That's my pulse after walking back to the exam room or infusion center and doing all that.

However, I still wanted to work my heart to a certain extent. I also needed to fit in my workouts into an increasingly busy schedule, including my full-time job. So I ramped up a calisthenics program at home, including stretching, compound body exercises like push-ups and abdominal work, and a variety of weight-resistance exercises with dumbbells. I split up exercises to work various muscle groups every other day, with Sunday being a rest day. And I put the exercises together in a circuit so I would jump from one exercise to another, keeping my heart rate elevated.

Of course, the emphasis on physical fitness at the start of my cancer fight factored considerably in the crushing fatigue I faced just a couple of weeks in. While exercise was a non-negotiable item in my routine, I needed to balance everything I was doing to make the process sustainable. I needed to be more aware of what my body and mind were telling me and take appropriate steps.

It became a tinkering process, as I was conscious of wanting to build strength and stamina and maintain my body weight instead of tearing my body down. I knew I would need my strength as my treatments progressed, and I wanted to put my fitness at as high a bar as possible, giving me ample room to slide a bit as my treatments escalated.

Exercise has always paid personal dividends to much more than my physical health. It helps with my systemic well-being—physically, mentally, emotionally, and spiritually. Those components all come together, working seamlessly, and they create a synergistic effect. I find I can't be at a high overall level of well-being if one of those areas is low. So I use one or more to help lift any area that might be lagging.

It's a conceptual framework that works for me, and I suspect it's something that works for a great many others too, whether fully articulated in their thoughts or not.

Chapter 5

HE SAID, SHE SAID

From the very beginning of my diagnosis with multiple myeloma, I've been overwhelmed by the gracious amount of love and support thrown our way by our friends and family. It's incredibly humbling to be included in prayers and to receive numerous messages checking on our well-being—not just mine but Lori's and the kids' too. I'm extraordinarily grateful for everyone and everything.

Thank you, everyone, for all your kind words, encouragement, support, and love.

From the start of my diagnosis and treatment, I've been inundated with requests. They're all a little different, but they're all variations of the same theme: "What can I do for you?"

You know, "What can I do for you?" is a somewhat frequent topic of conversation in support group meetings. Truthfully, I was surprised. Like so much about cancer and everything that orbits it, I had a simplistic view. The group helped me understand the various nuances surrounding the question of "What can I do for you"—and that they are as numerous as the patients experiencing a significant illness.

As discussed earlier, sharing a cancer diagnosis publicly is a significant psychological hurdle. It's not easy to come to grasp with as a patient, and I have to believe it's not particularly easy to cope with from the perspective of the person receiving the message, either. It's a shaky ground on which both parties stand, and more times than not, it's unexplored territory for both.

However, I want to caution all that the initial conversation—the breaking of the news, if you will—is just that, the *initial* conversation. There's this big moment of exhale after sharing a diagnosis, almost a sigh of relief, like it's "over." It's not though. It's just the beginning. And the next part too often gets kind of tricky.

In every conversation, there are at least two parties involved. And even in the best of circumstances, communication can be difficult because each individual is, well, different. Each party has their own set of filters, based on their values, knowledge, skills, and experiences. They have a message all worked up in their heads—or their hearts—and they encode that message by running it through their set of filters. What comes out is their blend of words, gestures, eye contact, and more.

Then the message floats over to the recipient, who hears and observes all these signals, and they then run them through their specific filters of values, knowledge, skills, and experiences to decode the message and take meaning from it. The process then repeats, and it continues, on and on. The process, people-based as it is, is rife with misunderstanding. Of course, that's nothing new.

At group meetings, I've heard patients express their frustration with hearing platitudes like, "Everything's going to be okay." Some patients feel a sort of anger bubbling from their frustration.

That frustration and anger often stems from patients just wanting to be understood and have their feelings accepted and validated.

Maybe the patient is feeling the effects of treatment or is tired, nause-ated, and scared. They don't want to be told, "It's going to be all right." They want to be acknowledged with something more along the lines of, "That must be difficult to deal with," or "I know you've got to be awfully anxious/worried/scared/depressed in working through this."

It's a challenging dynamic. For us, the patients, we are going into unexplored territory, swimming in deeper waters than we've ever swum before, and we are learning along the way. We don't know how to talk or act ourselves.

It's no easier for our family, friends, and networks. They're fre-quently in the same space as the patients, and for sure are in the same space with the patient in that one-to-one relationship. They, too, don't know what to do or what to say.

Yet, in the patient community, you still hear comments like, "You find out who your friends are." Yes, you do, both for positive and negative.

Some people will just disappear from sight and sound. There's a woman in my support group whose husband of twenty-plus years left her. Now, maybe he left her for other reasons, but she feels it's primar-ily because he didn't want to be along for the ride, having to face the extensive, all-encompassing, long-term cancer fight that lies ahead. Unbelievably, stuff like that happens.

However, it's my firm belief that those situations are extremely rare. More often than not, strained and threatened relationships are rooted in the levels of emotional intelligence of all those involved.

We, or at least most of us, just don't know. We should fess up and share how we feel, not what we think we know or what we think someone else thinks. We, patients and others, need to ask more ques-tions and listen. Together, people who genuinely care for one another will come out the other end with a stronger bond.

You know what they say about assumptions, right? When you assume, you make a [donkey] out of "u" and "me."

Ken Wolters, a cancer ministry chaplain who founded esperas-4cancer, tells the story about a female patient, a wife and mother, who was diagnosed with cancer. Almost immediately, her husband of many years made arrangements for someone to take over cooking, cleaning, and laundry, allowing his wife to focus on her health care.

His wife sunk into a deep depression. Over time, their relationship suffered, and their marriage became strained. Looking for help, they enlisted mediation from Ken. During a session, the wife confessed she felt as though her identity—her being the matriarch of the household, the supporting caregiver for her children and her spouse—had been taken from her.

The husband thought he was helping. The wife felt something deep in the core of her being had been stripped from her without being asked if that's what would help. Even a couple with decades of intimacy between them had let miscommunication get the upper hand.

Again, we, patients and others, need to give one another a break. Let's not be afraid to dig deeper into emotions, ask probing questions, listen with empathy, and have patience with one another on this difficult, unprecedented journey.

Miscommunication, of course, is only one potential threat to relationships. Another is fully understanding the needs of one another. Again, this was another interesting discovery I gained in group.

Jeff was a patient going through an arduous treatment program, and his sons were looking for a way, *any* way, to help. One son, who lived locally, wanted to drive him to his chemotherapy treatments. Jeff didn't want his son to drive him. One, he believed he could drive himself, and it made him feel good to drive himself. Second, he didn't want to be a burden to his son.

The thing was, his son's offer to drive Jeff wasn't solely for Jeff's benefit. His son was scared and wanted to help, but he felt helpless. Jeff didn't need the ride. But his son *needed* to drive him. In short order, Jeff recognized that, and he started accepting rides.

A lesson for all patients. Even if you don't *need* the help, recognize that others might *feel* the need to help. It's new ground to cover for both us patients and our loved ones. What do you say we give each other a break, huh?

As I mentioned, when I was initially diagnosed, I was bombarded with requests for what assistance could be provided by our generous friends and from my accommodating workplace. At first, I replied, "Nothing." Then, learning a few lessons at group, I put aside my reluctance and graciously accepted some assistance. Lori and I enjoyed a number of great meals from our friends—thanks Donna, Beth, Kimba, Chris Anne, and others and we didn't miss trying to squeeze trips to the grocery store into our crowded calendar of doctors' appointments, medical tests, and treatments.

Then, over time, as I was asked to speak to different groups and as I embraced the roles of patient community advocate and fundraiser, I developed a specific list of what others could do for me. For those of you reading, there are four important things you can do for me and for other patients.

#1—See your doctor annually

Go see your doctor annually for a physical examination, and as part of that exam, get a blood workup performed. And this is not a request for just you. Make sure you encourage your team—your family, your friends—to do the same.

Remember, my cancer diagnosis journey started with an anemic finding on a routine blood test—my hemoglobin was a little low and outside the normal range. That low value needed to be confirmed, and then I needed some expanded blood testing to determine possible root causes.

Here's why I want you to go to the doctor: From my routine blood screening, additional testing led to discovering that 90 percent of my bone marrow was cancerous. During that time, I had no overt, obvious symptoms. Sure, maybe I was a bit tired, but give me a break; I was fifty-four years old, working long hours at a startup technology company, and trying to get two kids through expensive colleges. During my workouts, I was crushing it, with my performance metrics on par, if not a bit better, than the metrics of the previous five years.

Cancer is silent; it's a sneaky little opponent that creeps up on you. One out of three Americans will experience cancer firsthand in their lifetime—some estimates peg that number at 40 percent, or four out of ten.[3] Rest assured that nearly all of us will undoubtedly have someone in our family, social circles, and/or networks go through a cancer diagnosis. Cancer affects nearly everyone, to one degree or another. Tell your team, spread the word, raise awareness, and lead by proactive example.

#2—Eliminate, or at least minimize, as many risk factors as you're so inclined

Minimize your risk factors. You don't need a doctor or any genetic testing, and especially me, to tell you what those risk factors are. You already know—I call them the "toos." They're the "too muches" and the "too littles."

You know, like:

- You drink too much
- You eat too much
- You smoke too much
- You exercise too little
- You eat too few fruits and vegetables

You get it. You know what risk factors you have.

I'm not asking you to stop living a joyful and happy life. That's ridiculous. What I'm asking you is to recognize your risk factors and minimize—or even eliminate—those with which you're comfortable. It will make for a healthier you, and a healthier you makes for a happier me.

#3—Reach out to those who are alone in their health struggles

If you know someone going through cancer or any other health crisis alone, please reach out to them. Let them know you're thinking of them and would love to help in any way you can. Perhaps even offer up a few specifics, like providing rides to treatments or other appointments, or preparing a ready-to-eat meal or two.

I'm super lucky. I have had Lori, my wife, by my side through my entire ordeal—every appointment, every treatment, every . . . thing, every day.

I can't fathom going through this daunting fight alone. As a patient, there are so many things that get dropped into your lap suddenly. The almost endless appointments, a bunch of medications to manage, wading through the quagmire of the American insurance system, taking care of your day-to-day responsibilities, and, oh yeah, taking care of your own well-being too.

For Lori and me, there's rarely a day that goes by that we don't get correspondence in the mail. I'm referring to old-school snail mail. We get a load of emails too. Just the correspondence alone from medical providers, pharmacies and pharmaceutical companies, and insurance companies takes an enormous amount of time and mental energy to sift through. Thankfully, I have Lori to take on the lion's share of all those responsibilities.

Speaking for myself, giving cancer my best requires me to be at my best, and as I stated in the previous chapter, for me, that's a complex system of physical, mental, emotional, and spiritual well-being. They're interrelated, and one has an effect on another, even for healthy people. How many people skip workouts because they just don't mentally feel like it? Think about all those New Year's resolutions to exercise broken by the end of January. Not because a person is injured, but because they just don't feel like it.

Cancer patients can't afford to not take care of themselves because they don't feel like it.

For me, particularly early in my diagnosis, it was an emotional roller coaster, with plenty of ups and downs. It meant everything to know that I have an army of friends not behind me but alongside me, and together, we're marching into my, or rather, *our* fight. Numbers count—at least they do for me.

My people help lift my spirits, mentally and emotionally. In turn, that gives me the strength and energy to exercise. Exercising energizes me, empowering me to go to the market, source nutritious food, and prepare healthy meals. That gets me set for doctor visits and my regimen of meds and treatments.

Reach out. And remember, if you don't know what to say to someone, start there and fess up. "I don't know what to say. But I love you and care for you, and I want to help support you along the way the best I can. I hope we can talk about how to do that."

It will mean the world to the person you share it with.

#4—Find a health cause; make it your cause

Find your health-related cause, whatever that may be. You'll know your cause when one calls out to you, for it will be the one you're most passionate about. And once you've identified it, support it the best you can with either your time, your financial contributions, or both. We're in this together, people. It takes all of us.

If you're inclined to donate to cancer organizations on my behalf, I am humbled and flattered. I've also got some suggestions, including:

- Multiple Myeloma Research Foundation
- National Foundation for Cancer Research
- St. Jude Children's Research Hospital
- V Foundation for Cancer Research

Chapter 6

TO WEED OR NOT TO WEED, THAT IS THE QUESTION

When it comes to cancer treatments, there are many theories and an abundance of opinions about options, from pharmaceuticals to nutraceuticals and almost anything in between. There are an enormous number of different cancers out there, and every patient has a truly unique circumstance—his or her own body. Despite all the research over the past century, treating cancer is still only part science and a great deal part art.

Some cancer therapies are mostly art, and depending on the attending physician—a mix-and-match affair of a variety of chemotherapy drugs, along with doses, cycles of on and off, and other considerations. Other cancer treatments are much more prescriptive, leaving little room for diversion in any way that will produce a meaningful increase in efficacy.

With multiple myeloma, the induction treatment is pretty cut and dried, black and white. The standard is the RVD regimen—Revlimid, Velcade, and the steroid Dexamethasone. For the majority of patients, the only real decision is to do it or not. There's not really a gray area.

However, with subsequent treatments after induction therapy, it mostly gets gray, and there's not much black or white, even with established protocols. Stem cell transplants are a good example.

First, "stem cell transplant" is a bit of marketing magic and branding—take my word as a marketing professional. When I first heard it, I thought, "Oh, cool, high-tech and all that, a cutting-edge therapy." Then I looked into it a bit more.

For my Stanford medical team, the stem cell transplant I would be considering was an autologous transplant, meaning I would receive my own stem cells, not those from a donor. My stem cells would be harvested very early in the process and then stored, frozen, and, if everything worked out to plan, reintroduced to my body later.

In a stem cell transplant, stored stem cells are introduced back to patients so that their immune systems can be rebuilt. Stem cells will make bone marrow, and bone marrow will, in turn, make red blood cells, white blood cells, and platelets.

Now, why do stem cell transplant patients need to rebuild their immune systems? Well, that's because they don't have an immune system, none at all, after aggressive chemotherapy treatments to treat multiple myeloma.

Stem cells introduced back to the body are the back half of the entire stem cell transplant process. The first half of the process consists of several hefty doses of chemotherapy. That chemotherapy attacks the myeloma cells, hopefully decreasing their numbers in such a significant manner as to get the disease to a more manageable level.

Unfortunately, in the process of killing myeloma cells, chemotherapy drugs also kill a variety of healthy cells in the body. In particular, one's bone marrow is completely sacrificed as collateral damage. With the bone marrow goes a patient's immune system, complete with any antibodies from vaccinations and natural body responses.

Thus, bone marrow needs to be reintroduced so that patients can begin anew.

So, you see, the stem cell transplant process isn't so much a "transplant" as much as it is a chemotherapy bath that will injure all internal organs, kill cancer cells, and completely wipe out all bone marrow and stem cells. The "transplant" literally takes ten minutes to reintroduce the stem cells and then three weeks for them to lay the foundation for a new immune system rebuild.

But I've digressed.

Back to the gray area. With a stem cell transplant, the gray area is with regard to timing. The objective of the stem cell transplant process is to get rid of as much cancer as possible, with the hope of enabling the patient to be on a reduced level of toxic medicines, so-called "maintenance doses." But if you ask three doctors when a transplant should be performed, you'll very likely get three different answers—there simply is not enough longitudinal data on patient life expectancy to have a clear, black-and-white decision.

Dealing with that type of ambiguity was difficult. It's relatively easy to make a binary, yes or no, go or no-go, type of decision. It's much more stressful—and even frustrating—to make decisions when there are so many options, all of which could be the right choice. And, of course, all of which could prove, ultimately, to be the *wrong* choice. However, through my fight with multiple myeloma, I have learned to tolerate this ambiguity. It's a good thing, too, because it's likely going to be that way for the rest of my life as my doctors and I manage this disease.

Gray areas in treatment are particularly prevalent when it comes to non-traditional, non-medical care for cancers. Many non-medical regimens are proposed for cancer prevention, despite the lack of sound scientific data. After a cancer diagnosis, many patients leap toward those non-medical regimens for treatment.

For example, some cancer patients swear by alkaline water, hypothesizing that cancer cells don't like alkaline environments. Others swear by the medicinal properties of the antioxidants in tea, particularly green tea.

For me, green tea isn't an option, as researchers at the University of Southern California found that some green tea compounds, notably the EGCG compound, appeared to actually block the anticancer action of Velcade. Now, I wouldn't want to block the efficacy of that drug, would I?

One rather non-traditional elixir I began taking, completely on my own fruition and without counsel from either doctors or patients, is unsweetened cranberry juice. Multiple myeloma and its various treatments tend to negatively affect the kidneys. In searching for foods that supposedly promote good kidney health, I found some people believe berries, including cranberries, to be a sort of kidney superfood. I figured it couldn't hurt, so why not give it a try, right?

It couldn't hurt other than the taste, that is. A visit to the juice aisle at any grocery store will present you with a wide bounty of cranberry drinks, including sweetened cranberry juice and a host of cranberry-blended juices. For pure, unsweetened cranberry juice, you'll have to look at the far edge, almost hidden from view, and you'll spot a handful of bottles. I think it's because of the taste, which is tart and absolutely unappetizing.

If I didn't believe, or rather, if I didn't hope that unsweetened cranberry juice was promoting good kidney health for me, I wouldn't drink it. As it is, I shoot down a big double shot of it with a grimace, much like a novice whiskey drinker might shoot back a couple of fingers' worth of Scotch from a tumbler.

Speaking of *acquired tastes*, what about cannabis for the treatment of cancer?

Cannabis, better known as marijuana, is perhaps one of the buzziest topics in the United States, and there's no pun intended. Market analysis of cannabis suggests that if it was recreationally legal in all fifty states, the industry would be valued at over $70 billion annually. Is that a lot? Consider this: it would be bigger than the United States wine industry.

That's pretty big.

However, nobody really knows anything about cannabis as it relates to health. Despite what you might read or hear preached to you by advocates, the efficacy of medicinal marijuana is one giant gray area, with no real scientific proof one way or another. Lots of claims; but no real proof. And for what claims there are, they mostly center on the treatment of symptoms, like anorexia, chemotherapy-induced nausea and vomiting, pain, insomnia, and depression, and not the root cause of a disorder or disease.

I actually started ingesting cannabis edibles before my diagnosis. I was having problems sleeping. It wasn't a problem of getting to sleep—after reading for a bit, it usually takes just a minute or two. My problem was, and to some extent still is, staying asleep.

Prior to my diagnosis, after about sixty to ninety minutes of sleep, I would wake up, usually feeling hot, and then I would have difficulty getting back to sleep once my brain started getting busy, thinking about all I needed to accomplish the next day or beyond.

Unbeknownst to me at the time, night sweats are actually a symptom of several cancers, including multiple myeloma. Now, if you suffer from night sweats, don't go jumping to conclusions. Night sweats can also be a symptom of having too many blankets on the bed.

And you're going to your doctor for annual exams, right?

Back to my sleeping issues. I wasn't going to address the situation with opioids or anything like that—not my style. So, after having become a bit of a go-to resource for retail media when talking about retail cannabis sprouting up in the United States, I decided to get a medical marijuana card and try it as a sleep aid.

Medicinal marijuana cards are no longer needed for people over the age of twenty-one in the state of California. They are still needed for patients/consumers between the ages of eighteen and twenty-one, however. If you're not familiar with medical marijuana cards and the processes to get them, let me tell you: it's a complete joke.

Medical marijuana cards are not about medicine and medical care. They're about revenue and more so state tax revenue.

To get my card, I called an 800 number, where I spoke to a physician's assistant. I told him I was having trouble sleeping and guess what? He suggested I would be an excellent candidate for a medical marijuana card. All I had to do was pay $35, and I'd have a card allowing me one year of legal, hassle-free purchasing of marijuana products from any number of legal dispensaries throughout the state. No prescription, mind you. All my "medicine" would be self-prescribed—the dosage, the frequency, and the type (edibles, oils, flowers to smoke, etc.).

Medicinal marijuana, legally, is just state-sponsored permission, not a medical prescription.

Anyway, I didn't particularly care, one way or the other. I thought I would give it a try and see if it produced the results I was hoping for, mainly to fall back asleep quicker and more easily.

I'm not a smoker, so I took the edible route. Simplistically, there are two parts to cannabis—THC is the psychoactive ingredient that gets you "high," while CBD is a non-psychoactive ingredient and the component many people like for treating inflammation and other physical ailments. You can buy products that are one or the other, as well as both.

There are also two general strains of cannabis: indica and sativa. The cannabis industry tells consumers that indica strains tend to be more relaxing and sedating, leading to its nickname, "In the Couch." On the other hand, sativa strains are more energizing and uplifting. To muddy the waters for the uninitiated, there are also hybrid strains that combine both indica and sativa.

I started with hybrid edibles like mints, chocolate-covered blueberries, cookies, and gummies, all of them with THC. I started with three mg of THC, then worked up to 5 mg, and then 10 mg. I wouldn't say I was ever "high" from a dose, but truthfully, I wasn't really awake to know. I'd take my edible right before bed, and it would take an hour or two to work its way fully into my system. By the time I'd wake up hot, I'd throw the blanket off, roll over, and go back to sleep. Cannabis seemed to work for me to get a better night's sleep.

I tried pushing my dose up to 20 mg, and I didn't really like that. At that dosage, I began to feel the psychoactive effects. Or, I'm pretty sure I did. After all, it's kind of difficult to think straight when you're awakened from sleep in the middle of the night.

One night, I could feel what I thought was this little air bubble going up and down my esophagus, and I couldn't think about anything else. I sort of obsessed about that little air bubble and how it felt. Kind of freaky. At the same time, I didn't know if I was dreaming or having conscious thoughts. That night, I swore Lori said something to me and I replied, but then she didn't continue the conversation, which was weird because my comment to her was ripe for a response, or at least I thought it was. Was all that in my head, or did it happen? It was all just a little too weird.

That episode made me cut back down to less than 10 mg a night. Until, of course, I tried 20 mg again to confirm my first result. And confirmed it was—with the same type of experience. It wasn't just in my head. Okay, maybe it was in my head, but you know what I mean. No more 20 mg nights for me.

So there I was, ingesting 7 to 10 mg of THC and 5 to 8 mg of CBD a night. That was pre-diagnosis of multiple myeloma. Soon after my diagnosis, however, my friend Paul shared with me a 2016 published study from a team of Italian researchers titled, "Cannabinoids synergize with carfilzomib, reducing multiple myeloma cells viability and migration."

Now, Paul knows his way around the life sciences, having founded and built several successful biotechnology companies. He stumbles across studies all the time that state something along the lines of, "We found something that we think worked, but we're not really sure why." What he really liked about this study was the language in the study's abstract: ". . . we also found that the CBD and THC combination is able to reduce expression of the $\beta5i$ subunit as well as to act in synergy with CFZ to increase MM cell death and inhibit cell migration. In summary, these results proved that this combination exerts strong anti-myeloma activities."[4]

The researchers used the word "proved" and wrote about the specific mechanism that produces a synergy between CBD, THC, and carfilzomib, a selective proteasome inhibitor drug marketed under the trade name Kyprolis, developed by Onyx Pharmaceuticals, and very similar to the drug I take, Velcade. Apparently, it's rare for such strong, definitive language such as "proved" to be used, and since it captured Paul's attention, it quickly captured mine too.

The study has been referenced a great number of times since being published in 2016—sixty-four citations by my uneducated count—and while there have been no published reports of human trials, there seems to be some promise.

Most importantly, there's really no downside. I won't get into the effects of THC on the developing brains of children and teenagers.

But, from where I sit, a fifty-nine-year-old with multiple myeloma and a brain that's probably developed as much as it's ever going to develop, the adverse side effects of THC and CBD are pretty limited. Legal pot is taxed, so it's expensive. And if I take too much THC, I might run the risk of giggling too much, falling asleep, or developing a nasty nacho cheese Doritos habit and all that comes with it, like Day-Glo-ish orange stains on all my clothing.

But if cannabis helps me fight cancer, then it's a risk I'm going to take. The possible side effects of cannabis are nowhere near the extreme of the side effects of many chemotherapy drugs, which can increase the risk of developing secondary malignancies.

Over the years, cannabis products have improved considerably. Early on, it was my experience that a great many cannabis edibles tasted mostly like what I imagine dirt and weeds taste like. Now, most products are downright delicious. So tasty, in fact, I'd recommend keeping them away from easy reach. There might be a temptation to dip into them earlier in the day and a little more often during the day.

I keep my edibles upstairs, next to the bed, allowing me to resist their temptation to consume throughout the day. For me, I'll just stick to a small maintenance dose at night. At least, as far as you know.

The day my diagnosis was delivered by Dr. Raj, she had Lori and I meet with Rachel, her physician's assistant. At that meeting, Rachel sort of gave me an onboarding orientation in becoming a cancer patient about to undergo treatment.

Seriously. I got a three-ring binder and everything.

The binder contained a bunch of different materials, listing out various resources in the community. One thing Rachel brought to my atten tion was a tri-fold brochure and an application for the Sandra J. Wing Healing Therapies Foundation. She instructed me to fill out the application for a $500 grant to use as I saw fit for complementary therapies.

Being a newbie in this whole cancer treatment business, I didn't know what complementary therapies were. But, being the dutiful student, I did as I was instructed and filled out the application. Then I went about discovering what Sandra Wing and complementary therapies were all about.

The foundation was named after Sandra Wing, a former cancer patient. During her arduous chemotherapy treatments, Sandra found a degree of solace in complementary therapies like therapeutic massage, acupuncture, acupressure, and guided visual imagery. However, she quickly learned that modalities like those are rarely covered by health insurance. As such, as helpful as they might be, a great many patients simply didn't take advantage of them because they couldn't afford them.

I received my grant and thought I would try a couple of different therapies. I'm not one to believe that acupuncture, for example, will cure my cancer. There might be others out there who believe that, and I won't for a second challenge them on their beliefs. For me, I thought complementary treatments might help with the side effects I was suffering through during my RVD induction treatment.

The high dosage of Revlimid was wreaking havoc on my skin, producing a significant rash over my chest, the back and side of my neck, up alongside my head, and down my arms. When I saw Dr. Wen-Kai Weng, one of my referral doctors at Stanford, right after he introduced himself to me, he asked, "How do you feel, other than the rash?"

I didn't think it was that visible and noticeable. Apparently, it was quite noticeable, especially for a well-trained, highly experienced professional.

In addition to the rash, my skin at the sites of my weekly Velcade injections in my abdomen was swollen, discolored, and, two weeks after an injection, peeling. On top of it all, the heavy dosage of drugs was messing with my digestive system, giving me a mixed bag of both constipation and diarrhea. I know what you're thinking, and you're wrong. A person can suffer from both at once. Well, maybe not in the same instance, but certainly day to day.

Last, I had a wicked combination of both fatigue and insomnia.

I thought I would give acupuncture a try. After all, what's the worst that could happen, right?

Now, I've never been a fan of needles. Ever. I was that kid who fought every single childhood vaccination. I required at least one assistant to hold me down. In my better moments, two assistants were needed. I clearly remember my crowning achievement in obstinate behavior. After being wrestled down and held, I said, "Okay, okay, I'm ready—just let me catch my breath here." After a couple of deep breaths, I relaxed my body, and the medical assistant relaxed her grip in return. It was then that I made my break for the exam room door.

I have no idea where I thought I was going. I mean, even if I had made it out of the room, and subsequently out of the office, where was I going to go once I was in the parking lot? I was seven years old. It's not like I had a safe house in which to lie low for a while.

Ultimately, it didn't matter. The door was a pull, not a push, and by the time I was there to pull it open, the assistant was behind me to push the door shut. Foiled again!

Anyway, I've grudgingly become somewhat accustomed to needles going through this whole cancer-patient thing. Still not super excited to get poked, but I was at the point where I could voluntarily consider acupuncture.

My mother, who passed away a handful of years before my diagnosis, would be so proud. She'd be incredulous but also proud.

Acupuncture paid immediate dividends for me. As a patient who was suffering from insomnia, I fell asleep at my first treatment, taking a nice thirty-minute nap right on the table. After several acupuncture treatments, I also tried acupressure treatments, and I found them very relaxing. I never quite dozed off during a session, but they certainly were stress-reducing.

I don't know if the treatments helped with my skin or my digestive issues. They improved gradually over time, so there was definitely a correlation. However, I can't say with certainty there was causation. Maybe my body responded to my drug regimen better over time.

While getting treatments through my grant, I was invited by the foundation to a get-together at a sponsor's home in Pleasanton, the town where Lori and I live. I got to meet a lot of the volunteers at the foundation, as well as a few other patients.

One of the people I met mentioned during our conversation that she was Sandra's life partner. It surprised me. I had erroneously assumed the foundation was a memorial foundation. That's where my headspace sort of gravitated to at that time of my cancer fight. But there she was, just twenty feet away from us, Sandra J. Wing herself.

As a cancer survivor, Sandra is committed to helping patients in our tri-valley area cope better with chemotherapy treatments. Over the years, they've handed out over one million dollars of grants to patients in our local communities.

These treatments help patients like me feel better. When we feel better, we feel more empowered. We have more energy. We exercise more. We eat better and stay hydrated. We're better prepared to receive our treatments.

Cancer treatment is part science, part art. The entire medical community continues to learn. As patients, we owe it to ourselves to try different modalities and see what makes us respond to our disease the best.

Test, measure, learn, adjust, and repeat. It's a mantra that can be beneficial in almost every situation, your personal health care especially.

Chapter 7

HAIR TODAY, GONE TOMORROW

When it comes to cancer, hair is a funny thing. Not often funny in a ha-ha way, of course, but funny in a much more complicated way.

A great many cancer treatments are extremely tough on the body. It's the weird thing about cancer treatments, the patient often feels better before treatment than during treatment, lending further thought to the idea that the cure/treatment is often worse than the disease. One of the many casualties—collateral damage, if you'd like—of cancer treatment is the loss of hair.

For much of my life, I had thought, "What's the big deal? So you lose your hair to save your life. Lots of people have no hair."

That rather callous type of thought was before I was diagnosed with cancer, and well before I met fellow patients in support groups and at other functions.

For many people, the thought of losing one's hair is traumatic. So much of a person's identity is caught up in appearance; just think of all the time we've spent checking our appearance, primarily our hair, before stepping out of the house or even leaving the restroom at work.

It's a big part of our identities, no doubt.

I remember my friend Tony, a gentleman of about seventy years of age, speaking out at group about a possible treatment he might undergo. He didn't want to consider the treatment, and the first thing he mentioned in his position on the subject was that he didn't want to lose his hair.

Then there's Gloria, a neighbor of mine and a member of the same group, who continues to avoid one particular chemotherapy drug for her condition based primarily on the fact that it will cause her to lose her hair and it would be permanent—as in, if she ever started that treatment, it would be necessary to continue it for the rest of her life.

I spoke with Lori and others on the topic, how people were hesitant to lose their hair despite the treatment potentially helping them, *saving them*. To me, it's worth rolling the dice. A small price to pay for killing cancer, right?

But I now realize diff'rent strokes for diff'rent folks. Particularly for women. Lori explained that seeing a bald man out and about is not that uncommon. There's natural male baldness, fashionable baldness, and then, of course, medically induced baldness. The thing is, you don't always know one from the other. You don't immediately assume a bald man is a sick man.

With women though, Lori said, a bald woman is quite remarkable and noticeable, like Gail Ann Dorsey, a wonderful bass player who played in David Bowie's band for twenty-one years. A bald woman is somewhat of an oddity, and it's not a far leap for many observers to assume that a bald woman is a woman battling a disease.

Who wants to be viewed as a person battling a disease? It's part of all cancer patients' identities, but most cancer patients don't want it to be the main part of their identity, something immediately assumed by people they don't even know or speak with.

I get that now.

For me, I was told I was more than likely going to lose my hair undergoing chemotherapy during my stem cell transplant. Okay, so I would lose my hair. But if I was going to do so, I was determined to do it my way.

My stem cell transplant was going to happen after my initial induction therapy treatment, a process that would last three to six months. That gave me time to "get in shape" for the rigors of transplant, a training camp, if you will. And what makes for a better training camp than a total focus on the work at hand—nutrition, exercise, etc.? Since I was going to lose my hair at the end of training camp (and I had so many better things to do in the interim), I let my hair and beard go. No haircuts and no shaves necessary. Like Borg, the beard had begun. Only, I added a bonus segment, that being my hair. The beard and hair had begun.

If I was going to do it, I was going to do it my way.

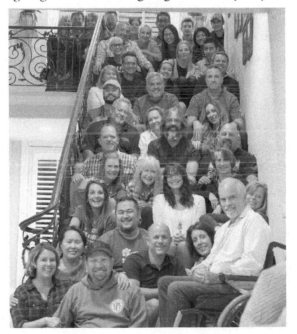

The author (center) gathers with members of his "team" to shave his head and beard.
(Photo courtesy of Tom Funk Photography)

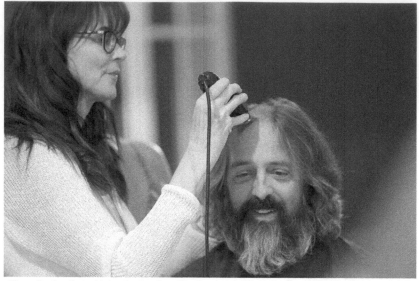

The author's wife, Lori, takes her turn handling the shears. (Photo courtesy of Tom Funk Photography)

My way was a shave down party just before my stem cell transplant process. As I guy who often had long hair during my adult life, too long of hair on many occasions, I knew I had a lot of friends who wanted their shot at cutting it off. So I offered them an opportunity—they could take a whack on my hair for a donation to the Multiple Myeloma Research Foundation.

$250 later, I was bald and beardless.

I was thankful I didn't have some weird birthmark on my head. That would have sucked. I was also immediately aware of how cold my head was, even though it was still sixty degrees outside.

By the way, having a shaved head is quite a bit different from having a bald head. With my initial treatment of Cytoxan (also known as cyclophosphamide and cytophosphane), the first chemotherapy drug I took during my stem cell transplant, I didn't lose my hair. Not immediately. I felt the irony of being in the small percentage of patients who didn't lose their hair after I had shaved it all off. I actually began sporting a bit of a five o'clock shadow.

Then, ten days to two weeks later, my hair started falling out for real. I noticed it first, I think, while washing my face. I literally washed off a good bit of my beard and mustache. Seeing that, I wiped a wet hand over the stubble on the top of my head, and it came back covered in hair.

Uh-oh!

I showed Lori and our friend Donna by rubbing my hand over my head four or five times, with the result being a paper towel covered with hair that used to be on the top of my head.

Going through the rest of the process, I lost most of the hair on the top of my head. I had some little peach fuzz on top, not new growth, but hair that just never left. Most every whisker on my face disappeared, save maybe twenty percent of my mustache and a thin line under my lower lip. I ended up losing about half of my eyebrows, and probably three-quarters of my leg hair.

Weird. Follicly speaking, cancer treatment had made me a naked mole rat. So I rolled with it, and had a little fun, even dressing up as Mike Meyers's character Dr. Evil from his trilogy of *Austin Powers* movies.

After all, if cancer was going to direct me down a road to baldness, I was intent on doing it my way.

One last bit about the shave down. In combat sports, like boxing and mixed martial arts, it's not uncommon for male fighters to grow a training camp beard. Shaving it off at the end of training camp is symbolic. All the training and hard work preparing for the fight has been completed. Time to pivot the focus from getting ready to competing and leaving it all in the arena.

In mixed martial arts, many fighters do a complete shave down, shaving their arms and legs to make it a bit more difficult, more slippery, for an opponent to lock in a submission hold. Just before the fight is also the time to do something about the hair, particularly if it's long. Usually, it's a decision to either cut it off or braid it up.

Again, the fight metaphor appealed to me related to my multiple myeloma treatment. I was at the end of my training camp, if you will, my induction therapy. I had prepared myself the best I could, taking care of my body with nutrition and exercise. I had attacked the myeloma cells with medication. I had prepared myself mentally and emotionally to step into the ring and force the issue with a stem cell transplant.

It was the end of summer in one heck of a difficult year. But I knew I was just getting started. The tough part was in the foreseeable future, not some far-off date. It was "go time."

Chapter 8

THE FIRST STEPS OF
THE STEM CELL TRANSPLANT JOURNEY

As written previously, the relatively standard treatment for multiple myeloma patients is an induction therapy of Revlimid, Velcade, and Dexamethasone, followed up by a stem cell transplant if the patient is healthy and young enough.

When I first heard of stem cell transplants, I thought about some high-tech process, what with stem cells headlines in so many stories for the past couple of decades, sometimes very controversially so. I didn't bother looking into any details about a stem cell transplant because, honestly, I didn't want to know.

My approach to almost everything is to focus on what I can control and let the other things kind of fall where they may. It's a compartmentalization strategy that helps me focus on what I think matters most at the time. And it's a great tactic for almost every project management scenario. During my induction therapy, I felt the need to compartmentalize my initial treatment, completely committing myself to the immediate task at hand, and looking to control, or at least influence, all the variables on which I could exert at least some control.

As I progressed through treatment and a stem cell transplant became the obvious next step, I started looking more into it. It was then that I learned what a stem cell transplant was and what I would go through.

For blood and marrow cancer therapies, there are two types of stem cell transplants. An autologous stem cell transplant is one where the patient's own stem cells are taken, stored, and then transplanted back into the patient's body after heavy doses of chemotherapy. No donor cells are required. An allogeneic stem cell transplant, on the other hand, requires a donor's healthy stem cells be transplanted into the cancer patient after the patient first undergoes intensive chemotherapy or radiation therapy.

With my multiple myeloma, I underwent an autologous stem cell transplant—not needing a donor and all that goes with that, in particular, any necessity for my family to undergo testing and the like.

I breathed a heavy sigh of relief when I learned my anticipated treatment would be an autologous transplant and that it would use my own cells. When I spoke to my sister Ruth about my upcoming treatment, she asked if she or any of her four kids needed to be evaluated as possible donors. The thought makes me shudder even today. I'm not sure how that evaluation process is done, but if it requires a bone marrow sample, I don't wish that upon anyone, much less a child in my family.

When I was first diagnosed, Dr. Raj told me I would go through my induction treatment for three to six months and then undergo the stem cell transplant. Being committed to being a cancer patient overachiever, I set it in my brain to go through the stem cell transplant in three months, in June 2019.

Then, in late May 2019, I spoke with Dr. Michaela Liedtke, a multiple myeloma specialist at Stanford. She asked me what my hurry was to receive a stem cell transplant. She said I might not need one at all, or at least not right away.

It was during that appointment that I was reintroduced to MRD, or minimal resistance disease. It was something I first heard early in my diagnosis, but I had shuffled it to the back of my brain as part of my compartmentalization.

Simplistically, MRD is the measurement of the percentage of cancerous cells. The most widely used standardized methods to assess MRD in multiple myeloma in bone marrow are multicolor flow cytometry and next-generation sequencing.

Patients want to be MRD negative. That means there are barely any myeloma cells in the bone marrow, and the depth, or extent, of MRD negativity in bone marrow correlates with improved progression-free survival and overall survival of multiple myeloma. For an incurable cancer like multiple myeloma, patients can sort of think of MRD negative as being in remission.

Dr. Liedtke saw that my blood value numbers were moving in the right direction during my initial induction therapy. Who knows, she suggested, maybe induction therapy would push my counts into MRD negative territory, thus eliminating—or at least postponing—my need for a stem cell transplant.

It was a possibility. Not a probability. I had not only a lot of cancer cells in my bone marrow to begin with, but I also had an aggressive form of multiple myeloma. Still, it reframed the context of a stem cell transplant, and I adjusted the focus of my care in response.

Throughout the summer of 2019, I continued to progress well through my induction treatment. My numbers were improving. My hemoglobin was within range, and I was no longer anemic. Despite the heavy dosage of both Revlimid and Velcade, my white blood cells were holding up, and I was able to undergo treatments as scheduled. More sophisticated blood tests as part of my myeloma panel were showing improved results, including a decrease in light chains (light-chain multiple myeloma, or LCMM, is a less frequent type of multiple myeloma, characterized by the inability of malignant plasma cells to produce heavy chains of antibody molecules, resulting in the almost exclusive production of light chains).

But, hey, there's only one way to really know what's going on inside the bone, and that meant another bone marrow biopsy. My second bone marrow biopsy was conducted at Stanford. Weirdly, just as the procedure was completed, the facility's fire alarms went off, necessitating an evacuation. Thank goodness that alarm didn't go off five minutes earlier, in mid-procedure. Just the idea of my nurse practitioner getting surprised by the alarm gives me the heebie-jeebies.

Here's about as good a place as any to get into a little more depth about bone marrow biopsies. Honestly, I've been kind of avoiding it as much as I could.

A bone marrow biopsy doesn't take long, thank goodness. Really, it's all over but for the kicking and screaming—and that might not be just an expression—in a minute. For most patients, the entire procedure takes thirty minutes or less, from the moment one walks into the examination room to the moment one walks out.

The sweet spot, so to speak, for a bone marrow biopsy is at the small of the back, where the hip bone extends to be, for all practical purposes, just under the skin. Step one is a local anesthesia injected into the area, designed to temporarily deaden the nerve endings.

Unfortunately, you can't anesthetize bone, and inside the hip bone is precisely where the patient's bone marrow will be retrieved. There's just no way of getting around it.

Well, actually, there is one way to get around it and that is with general anesthesia, a genuine option for small children. However, that's not really an option for bigger, older patients for two reasons. First, it's dangerous. While it's rare, one in about 200,000 patients die under general anesthesia each year. Second, general anesthesia is expensive. Your insurance company doesn't generate positive cash flow by paying out claims, you know what I mean?

Now, at the time of this writing, I've had two bone marrow biopsies, with more undoubtedly in my future. For my first biopsy, conducted in an exam room at my oncologist's office, the procedure was done the good old-fashioned way—by brute force.

I laid on my left side on the exam table, with my legs bent to be in a not quite fetal-like position. One nurse held onto my ankles in case I was tempted to move during the procedure. Then the attending physician's assistant pushed the needle through my skin and into the bone.

That hurt. A lot. Then the PA aspirated or withdrew a couple of bone marrow samples with light suction, from what I can only assume was a syringe. That also hurt. The rumor mill among patients is that the aspiration process is more painful the higher the quantity of cancerous or otherwise abnormal cells.

With that, the procedure was over. From the needle going in to the needle being pulled out is about a minute, I would guess. Then the site was dressed, and I got up and got on with the rest of my day.

My second bone marrow biopsy, the one that was to determine if I was MRD negative or not, was conducted at the Stanford Cancer Center, and that procedure was a bit different. Instead of inserting the needle by sheer force, the PA used . . . a drill.

Yes, you read that correctly. I don't know what the power drill looked like, as I didn't—and still don't—really want to know. But it sure fired up like a drill you might have sitting out in your garage, and, much like at the dentist's office, the sinister sound alone adds considerable anxiety to the entire experience.

Being a bit of a grizzled veteran of the biopsy procedure—literally, as my beard was at the peak of its powers—I felt like I knew what was in store for me with my second biopsy. As such, I really psyched myself up. I told myself that I liked the pain; I welcomed the pain. During the procedure, which Lori passed on by sitting in the waiting room, I breathed heavily, inhaling and exhaling through my mouth like I was ripping repetitions on a bench press. I was much more a steam locomotive than a passive patient. And I won't lie; the procedure hurt. But I gritted my teeth, worked those breaths in and out, and waited for the pain intensity to really hit.

After a bit, the nurse asked me, "Are you in pain?" It seems the procedure was completed, and had been for a little while, long enough for the nurse to wonder what was going on. Instead of the figurative kicking and screaming, I had been caught up in heavy breathing. I had been so focused on psyching myself up that I hadn't noticed when it was over.

That was when the fire alarm sounded.

Fellow patients have asked me which biopsy method I prefer. When pressed after initially responding, "neither," I have to shrug and say the evidence suggests I prefer the drill.

I can't believe I just wrote that.

Anyway, my second bone marrow biopsy seemed to hurt less. Maybe it was because I had endured the first one and had level set my expectations. Maybe it was because the aspiration process was easier because I had fewer cancerous cells in my marrow. Or maybe it was because of the drill itself.

In April or May 2023 (just a couple months ago at the time of this writing), I had a video consultation with Dr. Liedtke, and at the end of the call, I asked her if she felt as though it was time for another bone marrow biopsy. She smiled and said, "I would love to get a sample, strictly for academic purposes to see the data. But the results wouldn't change my prescribed treatment. So I would suggest it's up to you whether you want another bone marrow biopsy at this time."

Now, I do like academics, and the data would prove, at the very least, interesting. But as it wasn't going to change my maintenance treatment, you can probably guess that I chose to further delay getting another biopsy.

I might not be the wisest of men, but I like to think I'm no fool as well.

Alas, while the percentage of cancer cells in my bone marrow decreased tremendously during my induction therapy, I was far away from being MRD negative. That brought my medical team to a crossroads of sorts. Do I continue on with my induction therapy, or do I go through a stem cell transplant?

In my consultation with Dr. Raj, she used an analogy that hit home. She likened the situation to, of all things, a boxing match. I had my opponent, cancer, on the ropes, just barely hanging on. She thought it was time to go in for the knockout punch, winding up the ol' haymaker that is the stem cell transplant. Of course, that analogy spoke directly to me and my fight, *not a journey*, with multiple myeloma.

Leaning toward a stem cell transplant, I consulted with Dr. Liedtke. Reviewing the longitudinal numbers from all my test results since diagnosis, she, too, thought undergoing a stem cell transplant would be the best next course of action.

Thus, in September 2019, Lori and I started down the path of a stem cell transplant. We started two parallel processes. First, we made plans for that "End of Summer" party. At the same time, we made arrangements with Stanford for all the scheduling and counseling that's required for a transplant.

A stem cell transplant is a process, not a day. The actual transplantation of my cells back into my body turned out to be, in fact, a rather anticlimactic fifteen minutes or so. However, there was so much more packed into the before and after, and that was my real learning.

My stem cell transplant process was broken down into five distinct phases, one of which I'm still working through over three years later. Those five phases were:

1. Mobilization
2. Apheresis
3. Preparative regimen
4. Transplant/Stem cell infusion
5. Recovery of blood counts

Mobilization

To receive your own stem cells back, you first must get them collected, and that process starts with mobilization. You see, most stem cells lie back in your bone marrow, doing their jobs from the safety and security of home. And, believe me, patients most certainly don't want their stem cells harvested from their bone marrow. That would require tens or even hundreds of bone marrow biopsy-type withdrawals. Fortunately, there's a better way.

Mobilization is a phase that coaxes the stem cells into the bloodstream, where they can be skimmed off and stored for later use. For me, that meant a mean dose of chemotherapy and then a daily series of growth factor injections until I had enough stem cells in my blood to harvest.

But, first, I needed an easy way for my medical team to gain access to my blood, both for blood draws for lab testing and the easy administration of medicines. Therefore, after all my pre-procedure tests had been done—chest X-ray, extensive blood testing and profiling, and a urinalysis, to name a few—I had a Hickman catheter implanted in my chest during a short surgical procedure.

The Hickman catheter is a central venous line that makes access to blood much easier. During the stem cell transplant process, I had multiple vials of blood drawn every day, and there was no way the veins in my arms could have handled the load. Plus, the Hickman catheter goes directly into a large vein in the chest, and that's necessary for the administration of chemotherapy drugs.

The procedure to insert the Hickman catheter isn't much to write about. There's a presurgical washdown the night before and the morning of, and an awfully early morning at the surgical center. But the procedure itself is very short—two songs on the Pandora streaming service. Literally.

Terry, the nurse practitioner who inserted my device, asked me about my favorite type of music. When I told him hair metal from the 1980s, he found a channel. One AC/DC song and one Van Halen song later, I was being wheeled out. Terry and team gave me just enough conscious sedation medication that I couldn't remember the last three-quarters of AC/DC and the first three-quarters of Van Halen. I was up and out in no time.

The Hickman catheter went in high on my pectoral area, near my right shoulder. The internal part of the catheter was then snaked under my skin toward my neck, over my collarbone, and then down toward my heart and a large pre-atrium blood vein. There was a slight incision at my collar bone—I guess to help guide the catheter down—that was small enough to warrant just a steri-strip to close it. The hub of the catheter itself was sutured in.

The weirdest and most uncomfortable part of the Hickman catheter, for me, were the two lumens that dangled externally from the Hickman hub sutured into my muscle, like teats on a cow. Lumens are the access points to withdraw and inject, and they hang about six to eight inches or so. It wasn't uncomfortable for me physically, but mentally. It freaked me out a bit, and I stayed freaked out for the entire seven weeks I had the catheter.

After the catheter placement, later that afternoon, I visited the Infusion Treatment Area (ITA) for the first time. It was the first of many, many appointments there throughout the transplant process. That first visit was to get equipped with a four-liter bag of IV fluid that would be continuously pumped into me for the remainder of the day and night to begin a key hydration process prior to my initial chemotherapy treatment.

Four liters is a huge bag. *Huge,* I'm telling you.

So big, they put my bag of saline solution into a backpack and then strapped the backpack to a luggage cart. I had to literally wheel around a roller bag full of fluid, all being pumped into my freshly inserted catheter, tethered by six to seven feet of tubing. The roller bag, with its contents, was my constant companion for the next few days.

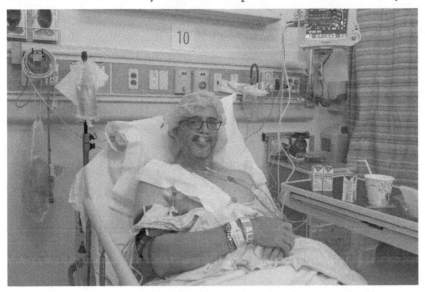

After a short procedure to insert the Hickman catheter, the author rests comfortably in the recovery room. (Photo courtesy of Lori Hartjen)

That night, Lori and I were too tired to cook, so we went out to dinner at the closest place to our hotel that we could find—a pizza joint across the street. It was a "last supper" of sorts, at least for a little while.

During a stem cell transplant process, patients are required to eat a low-microbial, or neutropenic diet, an eating plan for people with weakened immune systems. The diet essentially boils down to choosing foods and preparing them in a way that lowers the risk of foodborne illness. Because you can't control what you don't prepare, a low-microbial diet eliminates restaurants.

Pro-tip for those readers who have never worked in a commercial kitchen: If you want a healthy meal prepared in a safe environment, eat at home.

I've never felt as vulnerable as I did that night walking to the restaurant with Lori. I mean, it's not like Menlo Park, California is known for its mean streets or anything. It's quite lovely, in fact. But we still were out and about, and we had to cross a busy street of traffic. All the while, I was tethered to a huge bag of saline solution in a roller bag. And I'm not talking like I was tethered by something I had to hold in my hand, like a briefcase or something. Rather, I was tethered by a tube that was connected to another tube that dangled out of my chest.

I just felt so . . . exposed.

While it was good to get out with Lori for a date night of sorts, it was nowhere near the date nights we regularly scheduled with each other. We both had the weight of the stem cell transplant looming over us. Plus, the pizza was just so-so. As date night came to a close, we—the three of us if you count the roller bag, and I do—headed back to our temporary home, the Residence Inn by Marriott.

A stem cell transplant requires daily visits to the cancer center, namely for blood draws and an evaluation of what's going on with a wide variety of values. Based on the values of the blood tests, the patient then receives the proper treatment. For instance, a patient might be low in potassium, so potassium will be administered.

More importantly, it's an opportunity to check on vital signs—pulse, blood pressure, blood oxygen levels, weight, and temperature. The stem cell process wreaks havoc on the body's immune system. At a certain phase of the process, the patient has no immune system at all. Zip. Zilch. Zero.

As such, the risk of infection is extraordinarily high. So high, it requires the wearing of a HEPA filter mask anywhere outside the home or the cancer center.

Because of all the risks, patients are required to be within one hour of the cancer center at all times. In the Bay area of Northern California, that presents quite the challenge. At many times in the day, an hour in traffic can be just fifteen to twenty miles. Depending on the route, the distance between our home in Pleasanton and the Stanford Cancer Center in Palo Alto is in the range of thirty-three to thirty-six miles. However, at rush hour, those are brutal miles—a commute is an easy ninety minutes, if not more. And that's one way.

Not only would we not be within an hour to get to the cancer center, but we'd also have to factor in the commute home, and Lori and I both knew, on advice from my medical team, that I wouldn't be feeling very good the vast majority of the time. We needed to relocate from our home. Twice, in fact. Once for the mobilization phase and again for the transplant.

We needed a place to live, a place that was clean, had a refrigerator and kitchen, and had a private bathroom. More than just a room in someone's house as an Airbnb rental, we needed either an apartment or an extended-stay hotel room. And we needed it within an hour's drive at any time of day or night in one of the most expensive places to live in the country, the peninsula of the Bay area and the towns of Palo Alto, Menlo Park, Atherton, and others.

Needless to say, our living situation was a gigantic stressor for both Lori and me as we went through the planning process. We were uncertain if insurance would cover our housing expenditures. Actually, a couple of weeks out from the procedure starting, we were uncertain if insurance would cover anything at all. At the eleventh hour, our insurance company told us we were no longer covered at

Stanford and would have to have the procedure at the University of California, San Francisco.

Talk about stress!

Fortunately, our network stepped up big time. Paul and Donna, close family friends of ours for the nineteen years we had been in Pleasanton at that time, organized our mutual friends and raised money for our housing. Friends, households, and even children of our friends donated a night—and, in some cases, more than one night—at the Residence Inn just under four miles from the cancer center.

It was a blessing and a lifesaver for us—at the very least figuratively. It could very well have been a literal lifesaver as well. I'll forever be grateful to our team for stepping up and helping us out in a time of need. I'm absolutely humbled, still to this day.

Thanks to our friends, we returned from date night, crawled into bed, with me still tethered to my pump and saline bag, and tried to get a good night's sleep. We both knew that as far as we had come, the real journey would begin the next morning.

Day One of the stem cell transplant mobilization phase involved the surgical insertion of the catheter and the hookup to continuous IV fluids. On Day Two, things got real. Or, rather, more real. For me, Day Two was Thursday, October 3, 2019, and that was a day-long ordeal at the cancer center.

"Realness" came in the form of the administration of my first dose of proper chemotherapy, a whopping dose of the aforementioned Cytoxan.

Lori and I got to the cancer center early in the morning. As my Seattle Seahawks were scheduled to play the San Francisco 49ers that night, just down the road in Santa Clara, I came for my appointment dressed nattily in Seahawks socks and a Kam Chancellor number 31 Seahawks jersey. Chancellor is a former star player for the Seahawks, renowned for, among other things, his tough, physical style of play. I figured nothing could get me more ready than channeling my inner "Bam Bam Kam."

Our early appointment was required, as the administration of Cytoxan is an all-day affair. It was a beautiful autumn morning, and Lori and I strolled peacefully along the relatively short walk from the parking garage to the cancer center. However, as we drew closer, we both let our conversation quiet, and I walked a step or two ahead, focused on the day.

My nurse started me out with more fluids and pre-medications, including anti-nausea medication and Lasix, a diuretic that would make me urinate. Hydration and its corresponding urination are important in this phase because Cytoxan leaves the body through urine, and it can be harmful to the bladder. In fact, a fellow multiple myeloma patient in my support group was forced to skip the Cytoxan dose because he once had bladder cancer. Attendants don't want urine to build up in the bladder at all, so they see to it that patients are hydrated to the point of frequent trips to the restroom. Thus, the extraordinary amount of fluid and the diuretic, all in a quest to wear a path in the floor to the toilet. Because I would be getting up and urinating often, Lori and I were placed in a private room, set off from the rest of the infusion center, and with its own dedicated restroom.

Interesting side note on the Cytoxan urine: it's toxic. We were warned if there were any "accidents" in bed, etc., to shower and change the sheets while wearing gloves. Cytoxan is nasty stuff. My nurse wore complete personal protective gear, covering her scrubs, her arms and hands, and her face with a face shield when handling the Cytoxan bag.

That was for her. Looking at her with all her protective equipment was a bit disconcerting. For me, the patient, the Cytoxan was being pumped through my catheter directly into my heart.

Cytoxan took the better part of a few hours to administer, and I was able to leave mid-afternoon, once again tethered to a four-liter bag of IV fluids. Leaving the cancer center marked the beginning of additional safety precautions, namely the requirement to wear the HEPA filter mask in all hospital settings and outdoors and the need to strictly follow the low microbial diet.

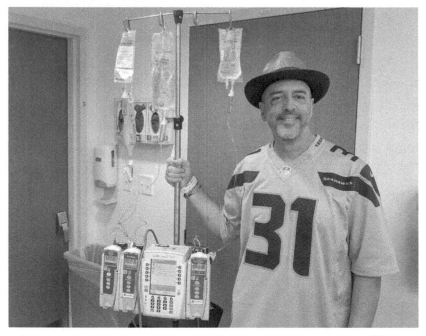

The author poses for the camera while receiving his dosage of Cytoxan as part of the mobilization phase of his stem cell transplant. (Photo courtesy of Lori Hartjen)

I had eaten a veggie burger from the hospital during the day, and I felt pretty good leaving the cancer center. Going into the evening, I continued to feel pretty good, and I even managed to eat a small meal while watching the Seahawks win their Thursday Night Football matchup.

It was after the game that I began to feel . . . less than good.

I was naive about the nausea I would face during chemotherapy. Hey, I'm a rock 'n roll guitar player, for crying out loud; I've had enough hangovers to know about nausea, right?

Wrong!

On one of our first days at the hotel, Lori and I went to the store and bought a few select meals and snacks to get us through our first stint in Menlo Park, through Thursday night and Friday, when we were scheduled to return home. Not wanting to waste either the food or the money spent on it, we purchased *exactly* enough for what we thought was needed.

Then I learned a lesson that so many chemotherapy patients had learned before me. When nausea came to pay me a visit, everything we bought became what I didn't want to ingest. Just the thought of trying to eat any of it made me more nauseated.

Unfortunately, it was 11:30 p.m. when that realization hit me, just as Lori was getting into bed. I moaned, groaned, and begged her to go to the Safeway grocery store down the street and pick me up the most old-school, tried-and-true of nausea remedies: ginger ale and crackers. Keep in mind, I was already taking a prescribed dose of anti-nausea medications, something I had been doing all day!

Lori returned, and I managed to drink and eat a little, undoubtedly to assuage some of the guilt I had in sending my wife out into the night. Sleep came sparingly, as I still had to get out of bed frequently to urinate, and my nausea just grew worse and worse.

Friday, my follow-up appointment was in the early afternoon, and Lori considered arriving late for it because I was finally catching a nap. When I woke up, we struggled into the cancer center. With chemotherapy nausea, everything for me was a struggle. I lay in the recliner and napped on and off while my blood was tested, and I continued receiving fluids and intravenous anti-nausea medications. Based on the blood tests, I needed to be administered some potassium, and that drip required some additional time. It was then that I was able to nap some, and it was also when Lori got trained on how to administer the three-times-daily injections of 300 mcg of Neupogen, a growth factor designed to stimulate white blood cells to enter the bloodstream. That's the real mobilization part of the mobilization phase.

Lori got trained on the injections as I napped. Remember that part about me being so much more comfortable with needles than I was as a child? Well, there's a big difference, at least in my mind, in receiving an injection and giving an injection. I wasn't—and I'm probably still not—at a point where I can give myself injections.

Most patients give themselves their Neupogen injections. They come from the pharmacy pre-loaded into little easy-to-use syringes. Kudos to Lori, a trained medical assistant, for stepping up and injecting her scared, squeamish husband three times every day for what would prove to be eleven consecutive days. Our morning appointments with one another weren't a lot of fun for either of us. Together, we got through it.

While still at the cancer center and fresh off being trained on how to give the injection into my abdomen, Lori bent down to give me a dose. Before the needle even punctured my skin, I moaned. Lori and our nurse, the same nurse from the day before, looked at me like I was borderline pitiful, explaining to me that the needle was nowhere near my skin. In my defense, I might have moaned because another wave of nausea was sweeping over me. Truthfully, though, I'm not certain that was true.

Finally, late Friday afternoon, I was sent home. Lori drove through rush-hour traffic while I sat in the passenger seat, a blanket covering my lap and a sickness bag—just in case—in my hand. It was an hour-plus trip of me just trying to breathe and not get sick.

I'm not one of those types of people who enjoy getting sick to their stomachs. Yeah, I know, there's probably no one who enjoys it, but there are a lot of people who handle it better than me. I've seen people throw up and then get on with things—you know, the old "boot and rally."

Not me. Vomiting for me is like a personal death scene, like from *Othello*. I fight nausea with every fiber in my being, and if I do vomit, then it's pretty much game over for me. Wrap me up and lay me down, for I'm out of commission.

Somehow, Lori got me home with the contents of my stomach still in my stomach. I don't remember anything else from the evening. I think I just went to bed.

Saturday, I struggled a bit early in the day but started eating soup by mid-day and felt much, much better by nightfall. Sunday was a good day, and it marked the passing of the nausea, at least for the mobilization phase.

Saturday was also my first shower at home after the catheter insertion. Daily showers are important to ward off bacteria and possible infection. But it's a time-consuming process and not very easy.

The catheter—and in particular the dressings covering the incision points—needed to stay dry. So each shower until the catheter was to be removed toward the end of November was preceded by a lengthy tape job.

Taping a flat area, like one's chest, is a whole lot different from taping an arm or a leg. To the rescue came Glad Press'n'Seal Cling Film. Before every shower, I'd peel off a big swath of cling wrap and then tape down all four sides. Then I'd shower, all the while anxiously looking at the seal to ensure the site stayed dry. Getting ready for my daily shower took about ten times longer than my actual time under the water.

After my massive Cytoxan dose, the daily regimen was the three Neupogen shots in my abdomen every morning and an effort to remain as active as possible, including daily walks. Anytime spent outside, though, required my wearing the HEPA filter mask. Wearing the mask is certainly not the most pleasant thing in the world, but it did afford me the continuous opportunity of channeling Darth Vader from the *Star Wars* movies and repeatedly muttering, "I am your father." It also allowed me to break free, at least temporarily, from the prison cell into which I felt my house had transformed.

Having to avoid crowds and not being able to go out of the house without the HEPA mask meant that aside from a walk, I was pretty much a captive in the house. I quickly learned that doing any time in prison would be really, really difficult for me. I felt a bit stir-crazy after just a couple of days.

Because of the variety of medicines I was taking, I was forbidden to drive, so Lori served as my chauffeur. On Wednesday, October 9, we took a little field trip to Stanford to get the dressing changed on my catheter, and that was a nice diversion. It was also a diversion of last resort.

Stanford's direction was to get the dressing changed in a sterile environment. Finding a sterile environment proved to be impossible. We were advised to go to a "wound clinic," but Lori's many phone calls came up empty. Doctors' offices weren't sterile, and they said they pretty much couldn't sterilize a room for us. Even if they could, they didn't have the sterile dressing pack to swap out for the old one.

Frustrated, we had no idea what we were going to do about getting the dressing changed.

Somehow, Lori, refusing to take no for an answer, forced our way into the Apheresis room at the Stanford Cancer Center. Although we thought we had an appointment, it turned out, in fact, we did not. When we showed up, they were a bit surprised. But they weren't going to turn away a bald man wearing a HEPA filter mask, now were they? Luckily, they had a chair open and one of the nurses made quick work of changing my dressing.

It was also the beginning of daily blood draws to see if I had enough stem cells in my body for apheresis. Aside from that first blood draw, my blood was drawn at the outpatient clinic at Pleasanton's Stanford Health Care's ValleyCare Medical Center, just a five- to ten-minute drive from our house. There, I was most frequently served by a phlebotomist named Olga, who was wonderfully proficient in drawing my blood. Completely confident in finding my vein, she cleaned, stuck, drew, and bandaged me in less time than it took to type this sentence. And I'm not really exaggerating.

Sunday, however, the outpatient clinic at the hospital was closed, and that required another long trip to Stanford for a blood draw. Little did we know that the commute was going to become a short-term habit.

On Monday, based on the results of my daily blood test, the Apheresis charge nurse called and asked if I could come to Stanford for a sophisticated blood test that only their lab could conduct. The reason was that my blood values indicated I was close to the level where I could get stem cells harvested. So we drove over to Palo Alto for a second consecutive day, at rush hour no less, got my blood drawn in no time at all, and then drove back home. A nice three-hour tour of the Bay Area's freeway network.

When we got home, I got the call—I was ready for apheresis, and I should be at Stanford first thing Tuesday morning. That would make three consecutive days of driving from Pleasanton to Palo Alto and back. Believe it or not, Lori and I were thrilled to receive the news!

Apheresis

I found apheresis, as a stage, exciting. At its completion, it marked the end of the "first half" of the stem cell transplant process. As such, it also meant the requirements of a low microbial diet and a HEPA filter mask for outside the home were lifted until the "second half" could commence. Freedom and restaurants! Normalcy of a sort.

Apheresis, as an event, however, is not exciting. It involved sitting in a chair, hooked up to a machine for five hours. Blood was drawn out through the catheter, centrifuged to separate it by weight and density, with stem cells segregated and pumped into a storage bag, and the "leftover" blood pumped back into my body through the remaining catheter lumen.

Once attached, there's no separating from the machine. For anything. I didn't want to suffer the humiliation of urinating in a bottle, so I was very diligent in managing my hydration that morning, drinking just enough in the morning, and drinking nothing for a couple of hours after being hooked up. I started hydrating more toward the end of the procedure and made it through the five hours. But don't let me fool you—urination was an almost constant thought in my head throughout my entire stay in the clinic. As has happened many times in the middle of the night, once the thought of needing to pee entered my head, it was impossible to get the thought to go away.

After my session, I wasn't quite in the clear. The laboratory personnel needed to count the stem cells collected to see if they had enough for two potential stem cell transplants. If not, I would have to return the next day, and perhaps another day or two after that, to complete the collection process. Luckily, later that afternoon, I received the call—I overachieved and had supplied four times the requirement for what was needed.

With that news, the first half of the transplant was complete. No more safety precautions like the diet and the mask, and no need to stay in close proximity to Stanford, like during the hydration and Cytoxan days. It meant a resumption of normal daily life—albeit one with a Hickman catheter dangling from my chest—and a rest period for my body to build up its strength until the second half of the stem cell transplant started, seventeen days hence, with the preparative regimen.

Chapter 9

DEALING WITH CHEMOTHERAPY-INDUCED NAUSEA

The reason I started blogging about my experiences with multiple myeloma—and eventually drafted this manuscript—was to not only document my story of fighting against cancer but hopefully also produce a set of resources for those who follow me into the fight. For those who get a multiple myeloma diagnosis, I want to let them know they're not alone, that others experience the same or similar situations, and hopefully provide some insights into how new patients and their caregivers might approach and deal with all that might be forthcoming in their treatment regimens.

As such, it's time to speak to chemotherapy-induced nausea.

During my six months of induction treatment after being diagnosed with multiple myeloma, I was on the relatively standard RVD protocol—Revlimid, Velcade, and Dexamethasone. Two pills and one injection that required an easy four-mile trip to my infusion center.

That's a big thing, by the way, that commute to and from my infusion center. I was, and continue to be, fortunate to drive a short distance to receive my treatments. Many patients are not nearly as lucky, some commuting upwards of an hour to get to their infusion center.

I fully recognize an hour or more drive to subject yourself to the throes of chemotherapy and an hour or more to get back home after treatment is an entirely different type of burden. Again, if you know someone . . .

For my Velcade injections, I went to the infusion center, the same place as everyone else getting their chemotherapy treatments. My treatment was just a single injection. A Velcade treatment is a "slow push" of an injection, something that takes about ten to fifteen seconds. That's it; it's really not much at all, particularly relative to what other patients go through.

Most of the patients in the infusion center are there for much longer hauls. A great many patients lie back in recliners with blankets over them, napping. Why? Because their treatments are two, four, eight, or even thirty hours long. Yeah, you read that last bit correctly, thirty hours. A woman in my group used to go into the infusion center for an entire day of treatment, then, right at the end of the day, she would be outfitted with a chemotherapy bag attached to a pump to continue the treatment into the night and the next day. The next day, she would arrive at the infusion center just before closing and the staff of nurses would finally disconnect her.

I once got into and out of my infusion center in twenty-nine total minutes—checked in, waited to be called back, got weighed, had my vital signs taken, had a CBC blood draw performed and analyzed, and received my injection once the CBC results came back satisfactory for treatment.

I might have cancer, but I know how fortunate I am. I really do.

And while nausea is a possible side effect of the RVD induction therapy, it never really affected me. Revlimid gave me skin rashes;

Velcade bruised and discolored my skin, and all along, I had fatigue, insomnia, and various digestive issues. But that was about it. Seeing what other patients went through, I made sure to keep my mouth shut about any of my "hardships"—side effects and complications—because, in comparison, there really weren't any.

My stem cell treatment at Stanford began my first real exposure to hardcore chemotherapy, that being my big dose of Cytoxan. From that very first night, I learned a lot. I thought I had known about nausea, and I thought I had prepared well for it. I knew I would be given a lot of anti-nausea medication, and I figured I would be able to work through any nausea that crept in.

I knew it wouldn't be easy. But I didn't know it was going to be as difficult as it turned out to be. It's based on that experience that I'm writing this quick and dirty guide to dealing with nausea, often the most immediate side effect of chemotherapy.

1. Just because you don't feel nauseated doesn't mean you won't get nauseated

The start of a chemotherapy treatment isn't really the start of chemotherapy; rather, it's the start of a strong dose of one or more anti-nausea medications that takes some time. For my Cytoxan dose, it was the administration of a couple of drugs that lasted an hour or two. So the start of chemotherapy is really a relative breeze.

Patients know when the proper chemotherapy starts with the changing dress of the nurse. Throughout the preliminary round, nurses are masked and gloved in the normal type of medical masks and gloves. Then, when the main event is introduced, when the chemotherapy medication arrives from the pharmacy, it's a whole new process, with the nurses donning a comprehensive personal protective system—a long-sleeved gown over scrubs and, depending on the exact type of chemotherapy, much thicker and stronger gloves that extend well beyond the hands, with a face shield to protect against any accidental splashing or spilling. Nurses go through the precautions of preventing any of the chemotherapy medications from getting onto their skin or their clothing, or in their eyes or mouths.

Yet, as I wrote before, we patients are welcoming the drugs into our bloodstreams. Just looking at the nurses can be a bit discomforting as we await the administration of the drugs.

Just a couple of paragraphs above, I wrote that nausea is often "the most immediate side effect of chemotherapy." A longer-term side effect is secondary cancers that develop later. Chemotherapy drugs are poisons, designed to kill or otherwise damage cells. Of course, the hope is that the chemotherapy does all its damage to cancer cells, but collateral damage most certainly occurs in healthy, regular cells in the body.

Going into my stem cell transplant, my doctor advised me that all my organs would be "injured," but that as they were healthy, they would probably recover quickly. For me, personally, I wasn't worried too much about possible secondary cancers. I don't mean to sound flippant—like I don't take the issue seriously. It's just that I figure I'll worry about those problems if and when they ever occur. Again, it's part of my compartmentalization approach. My first priority going through my stem cell transplant—and continuing now through my ongoing maintenance treatments—was to effectively deal with my primary cancer: multiple myeloma.

Anyway, the point of number one here is for patients to understand that they will likely feel fairly good initially. However, it's likely the combination of both anti-nausea medications and that the chemotherapy hasn't really kicked in to do its work yet. Not all chemotherapy medications produce nausea, but for those that are known to do so, it's likely nausea is just around the corner, waiting for its time to present itself on center stage.

2. Get started by combatting nausea early and often

There's no such thing as being fashionably late to the fighting nausea party. I've learned that you should address nausea long before you feel nauseated. It's like hydrating on a long bike ride during a hot day, where you pre-hydrate before you hop on the saddle.

Then you keep it up. You know, sort of like voting in Chicago back in the old days—vote early, vote often.

From where I sit, it's better to be *not* nauseated than nauseated, and once one's nauseated, it's a lot more difficult to get rid of nausea than to prevent it in the first place.

It's a lot like pain management. When I was going through a back injury nearly twenty years ago or so, I didn't want to take any pain medication until I needed it—when I was *really* in pain. It wasn't that I wanted to be a tough guy, although I probably did a little. Rather, I didn't think I needed to take pain medication until I was in pain.

Then I found out a little more about nerve pain. On a zero to ten scale of pain, with a ten being the worst pain imaginable, taking pain medication at a level of six or whatever is probably not good enough. Taking medication at a level of eight is pretty much worthless. It's way, way easier to prevent it from escalating to an unbearable level than to reduce it from an unbearable level. A nurse, and my wife Lori, both taught me that back then. Well, they tried to. I learned it through my personal experience, the difficult, much more painful way.

For me, combatting nausea was the same. Best to get on it early rather than attempt to reduce a nearly unbearable level.

For my initial chemotherapy regimen, I was given anti-nausea medication intravenously at the beginning of the treatment and throughout the day. Then I was shipped out with three medications to continue taking—Zofran (which was one of the drugs given to me throughout the day), Compazine, and Ativan.

The great thing about these medications is that they can be taken together, so you can "stack" the meds to get the effect you want. So, for example, Zofran can be taken every eight hours. But, say three hours in, if your stomach is feeling a bit iffy, you can take a Compazine (which you can take every six hours). After another couple of hours, five hours since beginning with Zofran, you can take an Ativan (one to two tablets every four hours).

[Pro tip on the Ativan: Place it right under your tongue and have it dissolve, delivering it super quickly into your bloodstream.]

In the example above, the patient has taken three different anti-nausea meds in a span of five hours. That's how one stays ahead of the game! It might not prevent nausea entirely, but it's certainly a prescribed best practice for success.

3. Have a variety of food available

As mentioned previously, ahead of my first massive dose of Cytoxan, Lori and I went to the store to plan out my menu for the day of and the days thereafter. However, the mistake I made was I planned it out too precisely. Never being one to want to waste, we bought the exact number of meals I thought I would need, and we bought the things I thought I would like—a couple of frozen meals that looked relatively bland, some hard-boiled eggs for a bit of protein, etc. I also brought some home-baked Anytime Bars from *The Cancer-Fighting Kitchen* cookbook and a variety of quick and easy protein bar types of snacks.

Here's the thing, though: when the time came to eat while I was nauseated, none of it seemed appetizing. Absolutely none of it.

I mean, I couldn't even *think* about a hard-boiled egg, particularly the idea of a chalky yolk, much less eat one.

What I discovered is that other than crackers, the idea of anything dry or scratchy on my throat turned me off. All that protein bar stuff—I wasn't eating that.

So I had nothing that really appealed to me and, as a result, I didn't eat enough. For me, there has always been a fine line between hunger and nausea, even without chemotherapy. Not eating at regular, short intervals led me to feel more nauseated, not less.

My advice is to have a lot of variety available to you. You likely won't know what you want—or even more importantly, what you *don't* want—until you're there, in the moment. Don't plan too precisely (e.g.; three specific meals for a day). Rather, have a lot of options in small quantities and food items that can be prepared quickly. You might like the idea of a roasted chicken, but by the time a chicken is roasted for you, you might not want it.

Some of the things I found I wanted were vanilla yogurt, canned fruits like pineapple, low-calorie ginger ale, Goldfish crackers, and hearty soups that took up space in my stomach, in particular Chunky's Pub-Style Chicken Pot Pie.

4. Eat small bites, often

Don't plan out three big meals a day. They're too difficult to make, for one. Second, you're probably not going to want them. But most importantly, it means too much time between eating.

If possible, get into a habit of almost non-stop snacking throughout the several days after a chemotherapy treatment. You're probably going to feel better with something in your stomach, so make an effort to nibble on something every fifteen to thirty minutes. It doesn't have to be a lot—one bite of something is so much better than no bites of everything.

5. Drink lots of fluids

Fluids are important post-chemo, and the good thing is soup is considered a fluid, so a bowl of chicken noodle checks two boxes.

Water might not be the best thing for nausea, though. Now, I love water. I drink water throughout the entire day, every day. But water does have a bit of a "dead" and/or "metallic" kind of taste, particularly if one's taste buds change during chemotherapy, which happens quite frequently to patients. I found a stomach full of water made me feel more nauseated.

Try adding flavored electrolyte solutions to your water, be it a powered mix or a bottled drink like Gatorade.

6. Add ginger and peppermint to your anti-nausea plan

There are a billion people on the planet who think ginger and peppermint both have great digestive properties. It's been the home remedy for nausea for centuries. Late to the game, I discovered the reason for their popularity. They tend to work!

As I have told some of my friends, chemotherapy doesn't suck. It's the hours and days immediately after chemotherapy that sucks. You won't know until you're in the moment, but planning to have a bunch of options readily available to you will put you in the best possible position to mitigate the common side effect of nausea.

Chapter 10

THE SECOND HALF OF THE STEM CELL TRANSPLANT: PREPARATIVE REGIMEN, TRANSPLANT & RECOVERY

To be completely honest with you, I've been putting off drafting this chapter. I mean, I could have easily drafted this chapter on the second half of the stem cell transplant ahead of the previous chapter on nausea. But I didn't.

I didn't because I was hesitant to relive the lion's share of the entire stem cell transplant process. Simply, it sucked. It was a long, arduous haul, and more often than not, I felt fairly miserable. I'd rather write about nausea than the second part of my stem cell transplant.

However, the time has come. So on with it, we go!

As you'll recall, we left off the stem cell process with apheresis. That one event, the five-hour procedure to capture stem cells, was a significant milestone for me mentally and emotionally. At the completion of the procedure, and the confirmation later in the day that more than enough stem cells had been collected for my transplant, I was released back to normal life. I still had the catheter in my chest, so I still felt a bit like a circus freak, of sorts. But I no longer had restrictions on wearing my HEPA filter mask or adhering to a low-microbial diet.

To celebrate, Lori and I ate dinner out at Mendocino Farms. I can't tell you the pleasure of getting to this degree of normalcy, to sit outside on a nice autumn evening and people-watch while eating a big salad. Together, we softly, and in our own way, celebrated one milestone on the way through the process. Now it was time to focus on resting up for the stretch run.

For me, the rest and recovery period was a chance to get my body and mind prepared for the second half, which was coming up in just seventeen days. It was a chance to walk, maintain my endurance and stamina, and get organized and prepared for proper coverage during a particularly busy time at work. Although, if I had known I would be laid off five months later as the COVID-19 pandemic broke, I perhaps would have spent a little less time on the work bit.

Also, it was time to pack! Just like with the beginning of the stem cell transplant process, the second half of the transplant would require Lori and me to be within one hour of Stanford's Cancer Center at all times, for three to four weeks.

Our days leading up to the second half were interrupted only by once-a-week visits to the apheresis lab to get the dressing changed on my catheter. It was literally impossible to find a local place in the East Bay area to do it, even at a hospital, where they had facilities for in-patient dressings only. We know several nurses personally, and they offered to help, but not only did we not have a sterile room to change the dressing, but we also didn't have the full dressing kit for anyone to use.

Frustratingly, Stanford seemed surprised by all this. As we began the process, we underwent a variety of counseling sessions, and everything was mapped out for us. The weekly dressing changes were just simple single-line items on an entirely full calendar. In the end, they were the most difficult things to arrange for logistically. In practice, of course, it was a straightforward, five-minute procedure that professional nurses could probably do with one hand tied behind their backs.

Be that as it may, we used the apheresis clinic to change my dressings, and it required Lori and me to experience the pleasures of a Bay-area commute.

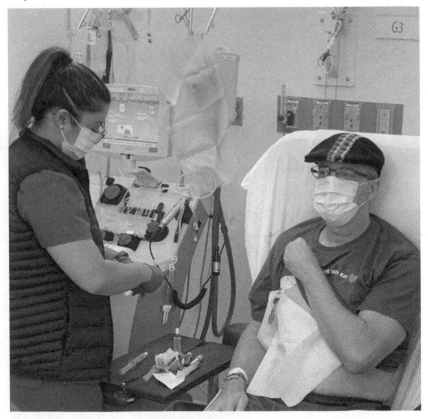

The author gets the dressing around his Hickman catheter changed by a nurse in the Apheresis Clinic. (Photo courtesy of Lori Hartjen)

Of course, during this entire process, I was highly discouraged from driving, based on all the medication I was taking. We took that seriously. I was completely dependent on Lori to take me everywhere, including appointments, and that dependency would only grow as we approached the second half of the stem cell transplant process.

With a whole host of preliminary lab tests scheduled for bright and early on Wednesday, October 30—chest X-rays, urinalysis, and a blood draw—Lori and I moved into the Residence Inn in Menlo Park on Tuesday the 29th and settled in for the long haul. Spearheaded by Donna and Paul, our connected mutual network of friends took care of our housing arrangements in September, and it provided Lori and me with a tremendous amount of peace of mind, stepping into this entire endeavor. We moved into a nice two-bedroom suite, with a kitchen, living and dining area, and two bathrooms.

However, as nice as it was, I would grow to really want to leave that place.

For the appointments on the 30th, what with it being the day before Halloween and having an overwhelming desire to insert some levity into my medical procedures, I decided to dress in my Opposuits "Day of the Dude" suit, just to put some smiles on peoples' faces at the cancer center. It seemed to work, too, so I wore the suit most of the day on Halloween as well.

Our daughter Olivia took some time off from Vanderbilt Law School and came out to visit for a couple of days. I guess she felt she needed to be there as I got started. I learned as a patient that I didn't necessarily need help and support all the time but that friends and family needed to provide help and support. It's what a patient's loved ones have control over, and patients just need to learn to say yes. As worried as I was that she would fall behind in her studies, I was grateful for having her around.

With Olivia in town, I decided a nice day trip would be to drive up to Baker Beach and check out its view of the bay and the Golden

Gate Bridge. I had never been before, and it was a beautiful day to take in the sights and be with the two most important ladies in my life. After the beach, we explored some of the city I hadn't been to before, and we uncovered a gem of a neighborhood pizzeria that, to this day, remains one of my favorite places to eat.

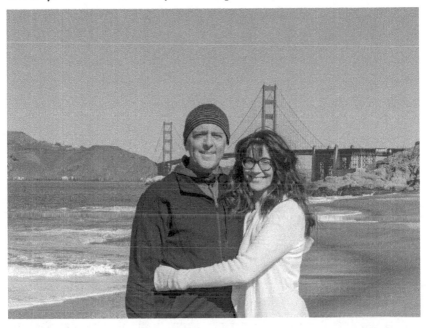

The author and his wife, Lori, strike a pose while visiting Baker Beach. (Photo courtesy of Olivia Hartjen)

Later that night, I covered all the bases with our direct family when our son, Raymond, attending classes at nearby Santa Clara University, met up with us at dinner. To tell you the truth, I can't remember what my last pretreatment meal was before I went back on the low-microbial diet—we were at a Mexican restaurant, but I can't tell you what I ate. I'm sure I enjoyed it, though, and I tried to soak in the enjoyment of a last night out before all the health and safety precautions, like wearing the HEPA filter mask, went into effect the very next day.

Friday, November 1 was the beginning of showtime. Another fight night, another game day. Olivia accompanied Lori and me to our 7:50 a.m. appointment at the Infusion Treatment Area. We got a nice spot with a good view through the windows and settled into a multiple-hour infusion of a proper chemotherapy drug called BCNU (Carmustine), a drug used alone or with others to treat several types of brain tumors, Hodgkin lymphoma, non-Hodgkin lymphoma, and multiple myeloma. The procedure was rather cut-and-dried, a normal day for the staff in the ITA, with the chemotherapy dumped into me via my catheter, along with a whole bunch of IV fluids.

Ah, yes, the fluids. Leaving the ITA that day meant another backpack full of fluids to take along with me, to be my constant companion for the foreseeable future.

The next day, Saturday, my sister Ruth arrived in town to help us out, and a huge help to be she proved. Not only did she prepare a number of meals for the three of us, but she also provided sisterly support to Lori and me. Also, importantly, she's a medical doctor, practicing emergency medicine in the Cincinnati area. It's always good for a patient to have advocates close by, and one with a medical background is particularly useful. That Saturday, we just had a single appointment at the Center, to change out my empty IV bag for a new, full one. Overall, I felt pretty good.

Olivia left to go back to school on Sunday, so it was Ruth, Lori, and me for my 2:00 p.m. visit to the ITA for the last scheduled dose of chemotherapy, a particularly nasty little drug called Melphalan. Melphalan acts on fast-replicating cells, like, for instance, cancer cells, as well as a patient's entire gastrointestinal tract, from lips to, well, you know, the other end.

With Melphalan, there's a particular worry of developing sores in the mouth and throat, a big problem when trying to ingest food and beverages. To combat that as best as possible, a patient undergoes cryotherapy prior to receiving the drug.

Now, this isn't the type of cryotherapy where people pay to stand in a pod of freezing air, or even the type of cryotherapy like sitting in an ice bath. No, this cryotherapy is decidedly non-high-tech. It's simply chewing on and swallowing ice, the intention of which is to contract the diameter of the capillaries and veins along the patient's mouth and throat, thereby having those areas receive less exposure to the drug once it's administered into the bloodstream.

For my cryotherapy preparation, I followed the procedure to the letter. While Ruth and Lori were talking, I was doing nothing but chewing ice and swirling ice cold water around my mouth and then swallowing. I dutifully performed my task for thirty to forty-five minutes. I definitely wanted to prevent, as much as possible, mouth sores. It's difficult enough trying to get medication, food, and water down under the best of circumstances during chemotherapy. Just like other patients, I didn't need any additional obstacles.

After the ice, the infusion began, and it went by fairly quickly. It was the quickest of the dosages, as I recall, but I can't seem to remember how long it took. Leaving the ITA that sunny Sunday afternoon, I was feeling good.

Unfortunately, that feeling wouldn't last long.

Nausea swept over me like a tsunami soon afterward. The Melphalan worked its way through me, and combined with my large BCNU dose from two days earlier, delivered a tag-team attack on my stomach.

All through the evening and night, I struggled with nausea, despite stacking my anti-nausea medications. Finally, I vomited for the first time in the wee hours of Monday. I threw up again later in the morning and generally felt horrible trying to shuffle around the hotel room, looking for anything to divert my attention from the constant nagging of nausea.

That's a difficult task for me, of course. As written before, I do not like vomiting. There's no "boot and rally" for me. I fight vomiting every step of the way, which probably caused me to think about it too much—those thoughts of "don't throw up, don't throw up"—which just led me to feeling more and more nauseated. After vomiting, I don't normally feel good at all, and it was no surprise that I continued to feel bad after those two episodes. It made eating and drinking difficult, and nourishing and hydrating are critically important for any cancer patient undergoing chemotherapy. Literally, every little swallow helps the body.

My daily appointment in the ITA that day was 2:50 p.m., so it was a long wait.

Once there, in addition to general fluids to keep me hydrated, I was administered potassium as my blood values showed a sharp deficit. The rest of the afternoon and evening was a case of hurry up and wait for the next day, for if all continued to go well—and the definition of "well" was relative, considering how I felt and my overall, general condition—Tuesday was to be Day Zero, or the day my stem cells would be reintroduced to my body.

Day Zero, My New, "Extra" Birthday

Tuesday, November 5 was transplant day! Of course, it wasn't the end of my stem cell transplant process, but it was a huge milestone in the overall process.

After the two most recent, massive doses of chemotherapy, my bone marrow was completely decimated, with not a cell remaining inside my bones. The hope was, and still is, that the chemotherapy courses did the same for the multiple myeloma cells.

Without any bone marrow, my body was producing neither red nor white blood cells, nor platelets. What I had coursing through my veins would be all I would have until either new, productive bone marrow was grown, or I had a transfusion.

I was still nauseated, but not as bad as before, and the vomiting had stopped, at least for the time being. Physically, I wasn't exactly raring to get to the ITA and start my procedure. Mentally, though, I was ready to take the next step.

The infusion of a patient's stem cells back into the body is a really big deal, naturally, but the procedure itself is a bit anticlimactic. Since my stem cells were frozen immediately after apheresis, they needed to be thawed. Then my bag of stem cells was added to the saline drip line connected to the catheter, and in they went.

There was one catch, though.

For their time in the freezer, stem cells are mixed with a preservative called DMSO, or dimethyl sulfoxide. Sports fans of the 1980s might remember DMSO as a sort of urban legend, miracle cure-all for a variety of joint ailments and inflammation. It wasn't FDA-approved for use, but that didn't stop athletes from sharing it in locker rooms. However, athletes soon discovered DMSO came with some interesting side effects—notably odor, both body odor and bad breath. You always knew who was using DMSO with just a couple of heavy breaths in a huddle. The perp was the one with "death breath."

Throughout my daily visits to the ITA, I would always set up in one of the infusion chairs spaced out in the facility. If any privacy was needed, there were curtains, but most of the time, we patients wanted to see each other, give a little nod of recognition, sort of an acknowledgment that we've got each other's backs and we're getting through this together. For the stem cell infusion, however, I was put in a small, private room, and I was seated in a bed.

The nurse overseeing my transplant told us the staff always knows when a patient is receiving stem cells because of the overpowering odor wafting from the room. Most of her colleagues likened the odor to tomato soup. She, I believed, thought it leaned more toward tortellini.

Now, I know what you might be thinking, but you're wrong. The odor isn't exactly like tomato soup or tomato sauce. It's "like" a tomato soup or tomato sauce, and the difference is big enough to be a notable distinction.

Within a minute or two of my stem cells being reintroduced, a smell of rotten tomato soup filled the room. It was plainly obvious. All of us—Lori, Ruth, my nurse, and me—seemed to adjust to it rather quickly, or at least, we stopped fixating on it. However, everyone new to the room presented a queasy face immediately upon entry.

I'll give you an idea of how bad the tomato soup odor was. Later that afternoon, Lori drove us back to the hotel, a trip of about ten minutes. Being in the car for just ten minutes made the car's interior reek for a couple of days. On Tuesday evening, Ruth ran a quick errand. When she came back, she said the car, despite me being in it for only ten minutes four or five hours earlier, smelled exactly like the exam room when my stem cells were infused.

I can tell you I haven't had tomato soup since November 5, 2019. I'm pretty certain Ruth and Lori haven't either.

When the chemotherapy treatments wiped out my bone marrow, they also wiped out my immune system, save the white blood cells I had coursing through my veins. My stem cells would, of course, be tasked with rebuilding my bone marrow, and, over time, my immune system would be rebuilt. But, for the time being, I had no immune system. At this point in the stem cell transplant process, it was a complete hard reset of my immune system. The day stem cells are reintroduced is called "Day Zero," and the medical staff refers to that day as an "extra birthday." It's like being born again, physically.

Of course, no birthday should go without celebration, right? As my stem cells were dripping into me, a handful of staff members helped us celebrate by serenading me with a rousing rendition of "Happy Birthday," complete with a small cake from the hospital cafeteria.

I quickly decided that if the cake was to compound my nausea, so be it. I cut into the circular cake and managed to eat most of it. To this day, it is the sweetest, most delicious cake I've ever tasted. Probably not literally. But figuratively, that cake's symbolic importance can't be minimized. Just typing this paragraph, I'm tearing up, overcome with a wave of emotion.

A big relief on transplant day was that I could leave the ITA without carrying an external bag of fluids. Ordinarily, on transplant day, I would have been sent home with a sort of fanny pack set up with fluids to pump into my body through the catheter. However, there seemed to be a shortage of some particular drug that was going to be administered within the fluids. As a result, my medical team thought I could do without any pump or bag.

It doesn't sound like much, but it was a big morale boost, and a welcomed one at that, to not be tethered to a bag and pump.

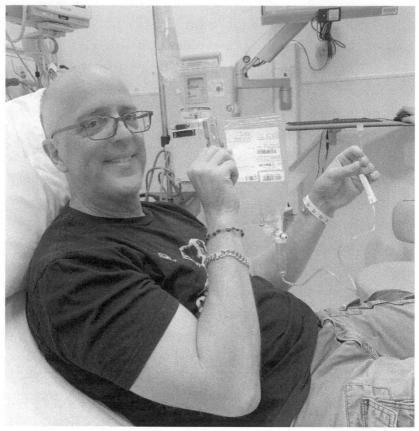

The author strikes a pose with the empty bag that previously held his stem cells. Thankfully, the smell of rotten tomato soup doesn't follow an image. (Photo courtesy of Lori Hartjen)

It had been a long haul, getting to Day Zero, November 5, my extra birthday. Looking at the calendar, it had been a touch over a month. But oh, what a month it had been, and it had taken a toll on my body.

We've covered nausea extensively enough. On top of that, and because of that, I wasn't sleeping well, despite being physically beaten up and exhausted. Then, there was my appearance.

The three big doses of chemotherapy had done a number on my hair, and I had lost darn near all of it. My beard and arm hair, including in my armpits, were pretty much all gone, as well as most of my leg hair. About half my eyebrows were still hanging around, though. But then there were a couple of stubborn patches of hair on my head that just weren't going to give up the fight.

I had this weird look going on, with dark circles under my eyes, no facial hair, two mangy little eyebrows, and a couple of patches on the back of my head. The nurse reintroducing my stem cells even commented, "I'm not sure what you have going on back there."

Losing my patience for my hair to fall out, I shaved what I could find. I only had to do it that one time. Soon enough, the rest of my hair fell out, and I was as smooth as a newborn baby, matching my newborn immune system.

After the reintroduction of my stem cells, each day developed into a dull routine. There were continued daily visits to the ITA, where nurses took blood to determine if any values were critically low and in need of supplemental treatment. Throughout the day, I tried to eat something, anything, no matter how small, even a bite or two, whenever in the day I could. I also consumed fluids as best as I could muster throughout the day and occupied myself with some work duties—all while trying to forget that ever-present nauseous feeling.

The cryotherapy ahead of my Melphalan dose worked fairly well. I didn't have mouth sores, or at least, I didn't have any sores that were big enough to be problematic. However, I did develop a sore in the back of my throat that made swallowing difficult, particularly when trying to choke down some of the huge pills I had to take morning and night.

I had a couple of pills that were about the size of my pinkie finger, from the first joint to the nail, but a little thinner. Ordinarily, it would have been a big chug of a swallow. With the sore in my throat, however, they just didn't want to go down.

Ruth, Lori, and I tried a lot of fixes. For some of the moderately sized pills, a pill cutter helped. When pill cutting still didn't work, we pulverized pills between two spoons and dusted them on a couple of spoonfuls of ice cream.

Eventually, it was a real struggle to get most every sized pill down. Efforts, performed multiple times during the day, usually led to gagging and then sitting still, trying to force myself not to vomit. Naturally, thinking about not vomiting only made me feel like vomiting more, and the cycle perpetuated itself, building in intensity. There were a lot of close calls—multiple occasions a day.

However, on Thursday, two days after receiving my stem cells, or D+2 in the parlance of my caregivers, it went beyond a close call. Several times a day, in an effort to fight off mouth sores, patients are required to gargle and rinse their mouths with a saline solution. I was homebrewing my salt water, and it was perhaps a bit strong. I sort of gagged on it and found myself fighting that vomiting feeling. I lost, and boom, there it went. An episode that put me down for a couple of hours.

In the ensuing days, my stem cells began moving into their new homes, my bones, where they were first tasked with rebuilding my bone marrow. Again, without bone marrow, no new blood cells are produced, along with no new platelets. Those blood cells I had circulating in my body were all I was going to have until the stem cells engrafted and produced bone marrow, and, in turn, the bone marrow produced blood cells and platelets. Ordinarily, that process takes ten to twelve days.

For almost two weeks, it's a game of wait and see for patients, nurses, and doctors. Lots of crossed fingers and hands pressed together in prayer.

During that period, my blood values continued to drop as, over time, my blood cells got battered about and frayed while circulating through my body, eventually breaking apart and dissolving. My white blood count essentially fell to zero—the lowest value the laboratory reports is 0.1, and I was at that score for days.

With no white blood cells to fight infection, I was particularly prone to any and all illnesses. Leading up to my stem cell transplant, I was weary of catching any illness that might delay the procedure. Now that I was deep into the procedure, my anxiety about falling ill reached a new high.

While my blood values were falling to their nadir, I started posting a slight fever and suffered through repeated bouts of diarrhea, in addition to crushing fatigue and constant nausea. From the medical perspective, diagnosing the cause of my fever and diarrhea pretty much covered the entire spectrum of possible root causes.

My symptoms could have been a result of my body's reaction to the doses of chemotherapy or to the reintroduction of my stem cells. Or it could have been . . . literally, almost anything else, both bacterial and viral.

With that, prudence required my medical team to place me on a strong antibiotic and then run cultures on blood and stool samples. The antibiotic came in a round pouch a little smaller than a softball, and it was connected to a small pump and my catheter for me to wear sleeping at night in the hotel. That was the easy part.

The collection of stool samples was far from easy. Of course, as I was fighting nausea, the absolute last thing I wanted to do was to start collecting stool samples of my diarrhea. It was another set of recurring low points in a valley full of low points.

To add fuel to the fire, my blood pressure started to get a little low. On November 13 or 14, my malaise was at its greatest. My energy level was as low as it could go, and it took all my strength just to get to the ITA Center that day. Once there, all I could do was lie around.

At that point in time, considering my low blood counts, fever, and diarrhea, the physician overseeing my transplant, Dr. Weng, decided to admit me to the hospital.

There was a challenge, however, finding a bed. At the time, Stanford was just opening its new hospital—the grand opening was scheduled a day or two away. In the old hospital, the Cancer Center had an entire wing for its transplant patients, but it was full.

We waited patiently. At least I was patient because I was too fatigued to get worked up about anything. I'm not so certain Lori and Ruth were so patient.

After a couple of hours, a bed was found, and I was wheeled over to the hospital and admitted. For me, it was comforting to know I was in the hospital because it eliminated the need to take my temperature constantly and then have to consult with the nursing staff via phone. There was a threshold level of fever that required a consultation, and I was always at or above that threshold. And the last thing I wanted to do was go back to the hotel, only to have a fever high enough in the middle of the night to warrant a trip to the cancer center and, possibly, admittance to the hospital.

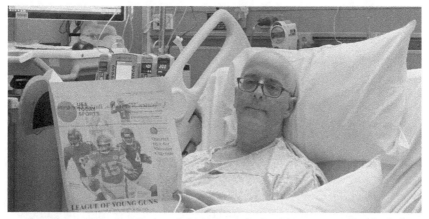

The author, catching up on the news during his hospitalization. (Photo courtesy of Lori Hartjen)

Since I could not be squeezed into the transplant ward at the hospital, I was placed in a room at the far end of another ward on another floor. It made for a long walk for my doctors and nurses, but it did offer me some privacy. Plus, being at the end of the ward, I was away from some of the hallway traffic and congestion that can be found with patients, staff, and equipment moving around. However, none of that helped with getting any rest.

For the first two nights in the hospital, I found it next to impossible to sleep. First, a nurse was obliged to interrupt the peace and quiet every four hours to take my vital signs. Those trips never really lined up well with needed visits to switch out bags of intravenous fluids being pumped into my catheter or for the administration of my many prescribed drugs.

Second, there were frequent alarms signaling a variety of errors related to the pump, like a bubble in the line, an empty bag, a kinked line, and the like. Oddly, in this day and age of technology, the alarm that went off was local. The alarm signaled the scene beside me, the patient, and it was loud enough to disturb the entire room. Where the alarm did *not* signal was at the nurses' station, staffed by precisely the only people who could do anything about my alarm. Thus, when alarms went off, I was awakened from my sleep. Then I would have to call the nurses' station to notify them of the alarm. A minute later, a nurse would come into my room and resolve the issue.

All along, I felt the entire thing was a bit ridiculous. I had cameras outside the doors of our home that could notify me, in a hospital thirty miles away, if someone was on my property. Yet, in the hospital, I had to call down to the nurses' station to tell them the alarm on my pump was sounding.

Through all the alarms, there were even more interruptions. On my first full day as an in-patient, I endured an almost constant barrage of necessary interruptions—the usual cadre of nurses and doctors, as well as a nutritionist and representatives of the hospital's finance and social services department.

At Stanford, the hope is that patients can go through the entire transplant procedure without being hospitalized. That's the goal everyone is working toward. At other facilities around the country, however, there are options for patients to consider, including having the procedure performed in-patient.

Some patients might prefer in-patient care if they don't have a strong support system, like a strong, healthy spouse or partner who can take care of them. However, when fellow patients reach out to me and ask for my experience and opinion, I make it clear that I found it almost impossible to rest comfortably and get sleep in a hospital setting. For that reason, hospitalization, for me, is a last resort.

Unfortunately, in my case, hospitalization was unavoidable.

After my first night in the hospital, Lori and I bid farewell to Ruth, who had to return to her home in Cincinnati. It was extraordinarily tough, emotionally, to see her leave.

Going into the transplant, Lori and I needed assistance and support, and when we did, Ruth was there to deliver. I was—and continue to be—extremely grateful for the time and energy she spent with us for those two weeks. I don't know where we would have been without her, and when the time came for her to leave, we weren't particularly eager to find out.

Fortunately, after my second night in the hospital, my fever abated and my blood pressure climbed back into the lower part of the range. I had dodged any serious infection, and that, alone, brought a big feeling of relief. I also thought I might be discharged from the hospital, and I was looking forward to catching up on my sleep back at the hotel.

Alas, my doctors had other plans. They figured as long as I was already in the hospital, they wanted to keep me there until my body showed proof of engraftment, proof my stem cells were producing functioning bone marrow, and that the marrow was developing healthy blood cells and platelets. At the time, I was still flat out of white and red blood cells. In fact, my blood counts were so low, I had received blood transfusions on two consecutive nights.

On days three and four of my hospitalization, I got up and took a couple of walks. I'm sure I presented quite the sight, fully masked with my HEPA filter mask, strolling through the hallways in my gown, pulling along my IV tree with bags of the various fluids connected by a tube to my catheter.

The walks gave me something to do and broke up the monotony of lying in bed. They raised my spirits. Lori walked behind me one day, taking photos and videos to share with the family, and I suspect those helped raise their spirits, too, after news of my hospitalization had broken.

I was trying to eat as best as I could, ordering from the catering service at the hospital. But eating was difficult. I had been nauseated for so long; I was of the mindset that everything I was feeling was nausea, including this odd type of feeling in the middle of my chest. The best I can describe it is a feeling after having eaten too much.

I was in a lot of discomfort, and it was so bad, I couldn't sleep because of it. Then, all of a sudden, seemingly out of the blue, a thought jumped into my brain: heartburn.

Now, I'm not a heartburn sufferer. I don't really know what heartburn is, but I've certainly been bombarded by television ads over the years. I googled heartburn, and I'll be; it sure seemed like that's what

I had, something I had ignored for two days and something that was just getting worse and worse.

It made perfect sense. After all, my Melphalan dose had completely destroyed the lining of my entire GI tract. That night, my nurse gave me a dose of Mylanta, and I felt it instantly coat the area where I had the most discomfort.

It was a proof point that you're never too old to learn something new every single day.

On day four in the hospital, my blood test showed an uptick in white blood cells and other values. That was a signal that I had engrafted, and I was set to be discharged!

After five days and four nights in the hospital, we were told we could probably go home. I mean *home,* home, like our house in Pleasanton. Out of a preponderance of caution, though, Lori and I spent one final day and night at the Menlo Park Residence Inn just to stay on the safe side.

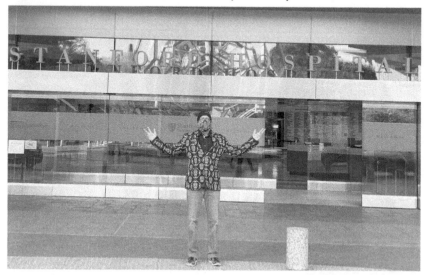

The author, discharged from the hospital and on his way home. (Photo courtesy of Lori Hartjen)

We got home on either November 19 or 20, the Tuesday or Wednesday before the week of Thanksgiving. All along, my goal was to be home for Thanksgiving, as that's my absolute favorite day of the year. In the Autumn of 2019, it was even more so.

I was still under precautions with my mask and low-microbial diet, but I felt myself feeling stronger, getting better, every day. When I had a follow-up appointment with Dr. Weng late in the first week of December, he advised me to judge my progress week-over-week, not day-over-day, as there were bound to be good days and bad days. When I looked at it that way, I could definitely see I was on the road to progress.

Overall, I lost fourteen pounds and went through countless hours of nausea, four bouts of vomiting, and days of just feeling crushing fatigue. But through it all, I found solace in being able to work for a few hours each day and play the guitar as well. And, of course, the numerous well wishes from friends around the globe really made a difference.

Revisiting the transplant to write this part of the manuscript was an emotional experience from the very start. I was overwhelmed at the remembrance of all the love, encouragement, and support I received from my friends, family, and community during that time. And to Lori and Ruth, the two who took care of me when I felt my very worst, I am forever indebted.

I don't recall the exact date of the removal of my catheter. Because of all the blood draws and administration of medicines, the catheter was an absolute necessity for the duration of the stem cell transplant process. But that knowledge didn't make me any happier with it.

I found it plainly weird having two tubes sticking out of one side of my chest like I was some sort of science experiment, which, in hindsight, I absolutely was. Then there was the entire routine necessary to waterproof the area before bathing. And weekly changing of the dressing around the insertion site.

I never got over the vulnerable feeling I had with the catheter. Naturally, I was in no condition to engage in a street fight or anything, but there was an additional vulnerability too. After having the catheter inserted, Lori and I were given a clamp, just in case blood started pouring out of one or both of the lumens.

Wait, what?

Each of the tubes themselves has little clamps on it too. Those would be disengaged before every flushing, draw, or injection and then re-engaged afterward. Over time, despite moving the clamps up, down, and around, the tubes had several pinch marks, and those were always very concerning to me. Once home, before having the catheter removed, I actually went to my local infusion center to have a nurse look at the tubes to see if any of the kinks posed a problem.

My catheter was a frequent point of worry, and it was an overt symbol of the process I was going through. Having it removed would be a milestone.

I often thought about the removal process, particularly wondering if I would feel it being snaked out of my body. That thought freaked me out.

Removing the catheter required a final, somewhat triumphant visit to the ITA at the Stanford Cancer Center—I don't think I've been in the building since (knock on wood). Lori and I happily braved an afternoon commute over to the peninsula for the procedure, which isn't particularly complicated.

I lay back on an examination table and a physician's assistant—I believe it was a PA, but it may have been a nurse practitioner—simply tugged the catheter super quickly right out of my chest. It was done in a flash, and no, I didn't feel it slipping out of my body.

I averted my eyes during the tug, and I didn't look over to my right where she placed the catheter on a tray. Just like with the bone marrow biopsy needle, knowing I might need another catheter some-day, I didn't want to freak myself out with the visual of what I had lived with in my chest for two months. Lori, however, took a quick photo or two for posterity's sake.

The PA put a quick dressing on the site and then a five-pound bagged weight, like the shot bags that can be found anchoring light stands on a video production set, to add pressure and stop any bleeding.

Through it all, my eyes filled with tears and my breathing caught with little starts and stops, while I tried to prevent a full-blown cryfest. Concerned, the PA asked, "Are you okay?"

Okay? I was better than okay. I was gently sobbing tears of joy. Removing the catheter marked the end of the stem cell transplant ordeal. Blessed and grateful, I was ready to step forward.

Chapter 11

THE INDEFATIGABLE HUMAN SPIRIT (AND HELLO KITTY TOO!)

Years ago, the buddies and I discussed the most ridiculous road trips imaginable. True boundary busters, like flying around the world for the weekend, showing up at work on Monday, and when somebody asked, "What did you do this weekend?" responding with, "Well, me and the boys decided to fly around the world, stopping briefly in . . ."

We let the around-the-world-in-a-weekend trip idea dissipate into the thin, fantastical air from which it bubbled initially, but we replaced it with another itinerary that squarely fit the bill for ridiculousness—flying to Australia for a concert.

Just a single concert. Fly "Down Under," hit the gig, and fly back. We joked about how we'd be cocktailing at San Francisco International Airport ahead of time, then hopping on a plane, whooping it up, and talking about how awesome it was, then watching a couple of movies, and then . . . getting totally bummed out, realizing we still had ten more hours of flying to get to our destination. And that would only be the halfway point of the entire trip!

We were going to do it, too, or at least I think we were going to do it, but the show we had earmarked, a U2 performance, was canceled as the Edge's daughter was going through a health crisis.

So back to the idea of around the world, right? My friend Paul and I ended up taking a modified version of that road trip in 2008. Not a weekend, but two weeks, from San Francisco to Honolulu, then Tokyo, Osaka, Dubai, Istanbul, Rome, Barcelona, Dublin, and back to San Francisco. It was on that trip that the legend of Hello Kitty, or rather *our legend* of Hello Kitty, was born.

We had a night flight from Osaka to Dubai, but when we checked in, we were told our standard-sized carry-on bags were too big to be accommodated. That wasn't going to work, particularly for Paul, as he wanted to ensure his computer and other essential electronics would stay with us in flight.

So Paul and I ambled into an airport gift shop to see what it might have in the way of backpacks or small bags. On the plus side, we looked for something other than a one-flight, dump-at-the-end kind of solution. Surely there would be something available that not only would suit our needs for that particular night but also something that would work for years to come.

Then we saw it. A unicorn in the midst of airport store sameness. A nifty, child-sized black roller bag with a nice, large Hello Kitty emblem on its back. We could use the bag that night, and Paul's two young daughters, Taylor and Kennedy, could use it for years afterward.

Paul quickly bought the bag before he could change his mind. But more than that, he immediately embraced the "majesticness" of Hello Kitty, dragging that thing around without a care in the world.

At first, I was a bit apprehensive about the bag. Oh, it was hilarious in the store. However, as soon as we left the store, I found myself slipping just off the pace as we walked through the Osaka terminals, sort of joining all the other passengers in watching the crazy *gaijin* pulling his Hello Kitty bag.

It wasn't long, though, until I welcomed the spectacular bag, first out of necessity, then out of just plain old fun.

I should take a quick moment and note that Paul and I have been, and still are, frequent travel companions. We have a blast traveling together, finding hysterical laughs in the most mundane of objects and circumstances. We laugh and have a great time. Others around us? Eh, maybe not so much.

Later in the trip, Paul proudly showed off the Hello Kitty bag to a couple of smolderingly attractive Alitalia flight attendants and asked them what they thought. One turned up her nose and said, with her incredible Italian accent, "It's for little girls."

Cracking up, we both shouted, "That's what makes it so funny!"

That Hello Kitty bag was the only thing we brought back from that two-week 2008 trip, save for great memories.

Fast-forward to 2019, more than a decade later, the year of my diagnosis with multiple myeloma. Paul and I had been planning another one of our trips, but this time, it was to include our wives, Donna and Lori. We were going to spend the month of September in Europe, the majority of it in one of my favorite places on Earth, northern Italy. We planned on finishing it up with a visit to Munich and the celebration of Oktoberfest.

Those plans disappeared in a hurry. First, there was the potential timing of a stem cell transplant three to six months after my March diagnosis, which alone would put the kibosh on a September trip. Even though it eventually turned out that a September trip would have been feasible, given my transplant timeline, the need to be seen in the clinic once a week for treatment made a month-long trip impossible.

With the Italy trip canceled, though, Paul, unknown to me, acquired tickets to see U2 perform in New Zealand in November 2019. He didn't know the timing of my transplant but took a gamble that I would be fully recovered and able to make the trip.

Now, I know what you're thinking. "Why travel all the way from San Francisco to New Zealand for a U2 concert when they'll undoubtedly play in the US?"

Well, that's simply not how Paul and I roll when it comes to watching his favorite band, U2. Together with Paul, I've seen U2 perform seven times, and only two of those occasions have been in the United States, and one of those two was in Honolulu at that.

Of course, when the time came, I was destined to miss the New Zealand trip, as I was right in the middle of the worst part of my stem cell transplant and its chemotherapy treatments. That posed a dilemma for Paul: What should he do about the trip?

Well, Paul not going to Auckland would mean cancer won, and we couldn't have that, now could we? In the fight against cancer, we tell cancer how we live, not the other way around.

As a result, Paul set his mind on going. It was to be a no-frills, no muss-and-fuss, down-and-back "road" trip, just for the concert. He committed himself to going to the show, for me, and to show cancer who's boss.

However, first, he needed to Hello Kitty up. The original Hello Kitty bag had been lost to time many years before. Luckily, a quick search on Amazon remedied the situation, as Paul procured an amazing white leather Hello Kitty fanny pack, conveniently delivered right to his door the very next day. He then stuffed Hello Kitty with a phone charger, a toothbrush, his passport, some cash, and . . . that's just about it.

Full commitment to the Hello Kitty protocol.

For a guy traveling halfway around the world, the Hello Kitty fanny pack turned into quite the conversation starter. I guess in hindsight, it was destined to serve that role, right? After all, what's the deal with a full-grown man wearing a Hello Kitty fanny pack?

To Paul, those conversations with strangers turned out to be the most important purpose of the fanny pack: the remembrance of two friends taking a big trip and, more importantly, the promise of taking more trips together in the future. However, those conversations didn't turn out to be just about Paul, or even Paul and me. In turn, those conversations experienced by Paul led to the commonality of shared stories and experiences across humanity.

It started on the plane to New Zealand, where Paul met a cancer survivor right across the aisle from him who had been through a transplant and was living her best life. Her advice to me, for Paul to pass along, was to simply follow my doctor's prescribed regimen to the letter and live healthily.

All along Paul's quick trip, people wanted to know his story and wanted to learn more. And word spread.

After landing in Auckland, Paul took a long cab ride to his hotel to rest up ahead of the concert, and, along the way, struck up a conversation with the cab driver. Side note: For you U2 fans, Paul's taxi passed One Tree Hill off in the distance—a fitting omen, don't you think?

Anyway, after a quick nap at the pool and a shower in his room, Paul set off, this time without Hello Kitty, to the bar for a cocktail before heading off to the show. Sitting at the bar, Paul, rather typically, struck up a conversation with another patron. Before long, the guy said, "Wait a second. You're that fanny pack guy, aren't you?"

It seems Paul's cab driver traded his taxi in for a bus after his shift, and he had shared Paul's story with an entire busload of Australian concertgoers on holiday in New Zealand. Everybody at the bar already knew of Paul and his story before he walked in.

It didn't just end there, with the sharing of stories. People looked to help in whatever way they could. After the concert, one VIP concertgoer gave Paul his commemorative U2 *Joshua Tree* 35th anniversary LP to bring back and give to me. Another, an Australian artist, told Paul she was going to complete a painting in my honor. Yet another insisted Paul bring back a New Zealand All Blacks rugby jersey for me, his reasoning being that one can't go all the way to New Zealand and not bring back an All Blacks jersey, right?

After Paul's down-and-back trip, he visited us at our temporary housing in Menlo Park. While his trip required a lot of time, and I do mean *a lot*, on an airplane, his jet lag wasn't too problematic. It seems from the West Coast of the US, the length of the trip sort of offsets the time zone differences. A quick oceanic road trip is actually quite feasible if you're comfortable sitting on an airplane for most of the day.

Paul showed up at the hotel bearing gifts. I received a ticket stub, an album, an All Blacks jersey, and, naturally, an authentic, "game-worn" Hello Kitty fanny pack. Plus, he shared a special video diary of his trip—you can watch it at www.youtube.com/watch?v=3IpBsjWIpII. The background music in the video is, of course, a live version of U2's "One Tree Hill."

I got a lot more than that too.

When I needed a morale boost, Paul and his experiences gifted me with a reminder of how inspirational the human spirit can be. To a person, we're so much more similar to one another than different, and all it takes to discover that is an authentic openness to engage, listen, understand, and empathize. And it only takes a few minutes too.

Paul's trip gave me a reminder when I needed it most, a figurative slap in the face. Cancer's not the end, not for me. Far from it. Moreover, in many respects, cancer serves as just the beginning.

I've come to realize that cancer doesn't bring with it the fear of dying. Rather, it brings the fear of not living while being alive.

The human spirit rises above all. The Dalai Lama has said humans are born to die. Far from me to argue with his holiness, but I say we're born to live, born to do. With that, look out for Hello Kitty to cross paths with you and yours while she and I spread the good word!

I'll be forever grateful to Paul for the many things he has done for me, my family, and our friends over the years. His visit with us during the transplant, along with his stories and the symbolic Hello Kitty bag will stay with me forever. Thank you, Paul. Thank you for bringing me along with you, in spirit, and for bringing back even more. I love you, brother.

In January 2020, Paul and Donna, as they often do, hosted a small get-together at their Pleasanton home. That night, Paul presented to me a wonderful painting, "In the Hands of Love, Joshua Tree," by the talented Australian painter Rebecca Collett, the very same artist Paul met on his trip.

The painting is strikingly beautiful, both in color and texture. It's another shining example of the love and compassion of the human spirit. Thank you, Rebecca and Paul! It hangs to this day in a prominent place in our home.

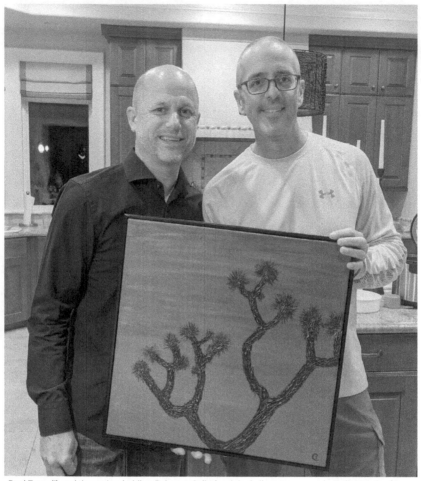

Paul Truex (l) and the author holding Rebecca Collet's original oil on canvas work, *In the Hands of Love, Joshua Tree.* (Photo courtesy of Lori Hartjen)

Rebecca is more than an artist, as she's also quite an accomplished freelance webmaster for a portfolio of clients. She's so talented that Paul contracts with her for digital work with his latest company, Thryv Therapeutics Inc., a life sciences start-up headquartered in Montreal.

I've helped Paul and Thryv on several occasions over the past few years, and by doing so, I've met with Rebecca several times, albeit virtually over Zoom video calls. We've come full circle. The world is an increasingly small place, although, in the drolly delivered words of famed comedian Steven Wright, "I wouldn't want to have to paint it." I encourage you to look up Rebecca online and check out her wonderful works on her website.

Although without our wives, Paul and I did make it to northern Italy. Because I was on a maintenance treatment program, it wasn't a month-long trek, but it sure served to salve the wounds of canceling our 2019 trip.

In September 2021, we attended the Formula One Italian Grand Prix at "the temple of speed," Monza. Naturally, Hello Kitty made the trip. In the relatively rarified air in the Paddock Club above the garages at Monza, I was the only one sporting a Hello Kitty fanny pack. In fact, I would wager I was the only one wearing such a magical utility bag on the entire grounds.

Oh, and it felt so good.

Chapter 12

WHO'S BURIED IN TAKEN FOR GRANTED'S TOMB?

Prior to my cancer diagnosis, I took a lot of things for granted. Looking back now, I can say with certainty that I took relationships for granted, darn near all of them. Truthfully, maybe actually all of them. The thought of a person might cross my mind, but I rarely took the action to reach out to them, inquire as to their well-being, and just let them know I was thinking about them. That was with the convenience of phone calls, text messaging, and emails, no less.

A letter or a greeting card? Forget about it.

It wasn't that I was purposefully neglecting my relationships. It was more that I was procrastinating under the mistaken impression that there was always time to be had.

Perhaps the root of my taking relationships for granted was my taking of time itself for granted. I took every tomorrow for granted, and a great number of next weeks, next months, and next years. Heck, I sometimes took *decades* for granted.

I lived with the idea that someday, I will . . . do whatever. Anything. Everything.

I don't think I'm special in falling prey to the temptation of taking time for granted. I suspect it's common for the majority of us, a part of our shared human condition.

On the road to my diagnosis, through the weeks of escalated testing, I went through a great deal of introspection. It was more than just facing an unknown illness and a murky, unknown prognosis. Who was I as a person? Who was the person I wanted to be? What had I accomplished on this wonderful planet of ours? What did I want to accomplish? With whom did I want to share? What was the life I was living and how did that differ from the life I wanted to be living?

In many ways, it was overwhelming. But, all the while, I had the realization there was an end to my finite timeline, and that end was probably a heck of a lot sooner than I realized just a few months before.

In my readings, I've discovered that some cancer patients have, over time, learned to view their diagnosis day as the best day of their lives. It's the day they started to truly live, recognizing that life is precious, and nary a moment should be wasted. Rather than cram their days chock full of minutiae, they instead look to fill their hours with what they're most passionate about, and with love and gratitude.

I'm not quite there yet with regard to stating March 11, 2019, was the best day of my life. All things considered, I'd have been pleased as punch if someone had just pulled me aside and said, "Wake up, man! You've got the gift of life. Live for the present and soak it all in."

Alas, no philosophical guru pulled me aside. Rather, I got the message, eventually, through my diagnosis. In quick order, it kind of snapped me into what I hope is a better version of me.

Many times in group, we'll have a discussion about what cancer has taken away from us as patients. Sometimes, it's disguised a bit, as perhaps someone framing the discussion in the form of "How has cancer changed you?" But, as the discussion starts, it's soon apparent that most fixate on what cancer has taken away. It starts with good health, of course, and then continues from there.

I fully recognize that my fellow patients are not wrong about feeling that way. It's what they genuinely feel, and that's okay. We each have our journey or fight, and we decide for ourselves how that plays out.

However, at times, those group discussions threaten to spiral out of control, and in trying to be a good, empathetic group member, I force myself to listen and seek to understand. On many occasions, though, these discussions have tried my patience.

I try not to be Mr. Rose Colored Glasses, but I've always been convinced of the power of positive thought. At the very least, it just makes me *feel* better thinking positively rather than dwelling on the negative. More than that, I actually believe there are good health benefits from doing so.

Not all clouds have silver linings, of that I'm fully aware. But I'm also aware that each action has an equal and opposite reaction.

Somewhat contrary to the group's general thoughts, when it comes to my turn to speak on the subject, I agree that cancer changes a lot. But I stress that, with apologies to Job, who is credited in his namesake book in the Bible, Chapter 1, verse 21, with writing, "The Lord gave, and the Lord hath taken away," cancer may take, but it gives in return.

I look back on all the roles I played prior to my diagnosis, which included husband, father, son, brother, uncle, nephew, bandmate, teammate, boss, and more. In each one of those roles, I had responsibilities for which I was accountable, and I had goals and aspirations I wanted to achieve within those roles. I might have had varying degrees of commitment to working toward those responsibilities, goals, and aspirations because of my habit of taking too much for granted, but nonetheless, I still had them.

And you know what? I still have them.

Cancer has done its share of taking from me. For instance, I'm somewhat tethered to an infusion center and regular treatments, so any idea of hopping on a sailboat and spending months at sea, traversing the world, needs to be dashed. Then again, I don't know how to sail.

With respect to my roles, I still carry all those roles I had prior to my diagnosis. But with my diagnosis, I've added more roles. Not only am I a cancer patient, but I'm also a cancer patient advocate, a fundraiser for cancer treatment and research organizations, a resource for cancer patients whose fights follow mine, and more.

Cancer has taken part of my life away; I'll grant you that. But cancer has given me much more than it has taken from me.

That said, March 11, 2019, is still not what I consider the best day of my life.

However, that day was an important day in reshaping the life I was living, and not just from health and medical treatment perspectives. Cancer has spurred me to spend more time with the people who matter most and perform the tasks that not only matter the most but are also most satisfying for me.

With my diagnosis, I took to ideating mottos. Not only do they look good on the back of Chronic Padres band T-shirts; but they also help sustain my inspiration and motivation. First, there was *Better Than Yesterday.* Then came *If Not Now, When?* Next, there was *Punch Today in the Face.*

If Not Now, When? tackles my procrastination, and my taking of future time for granted. Tomorrow's not promised, not for any of us.

So I ask you, if tomorrow is not promised, what are you going to do today? I use *If Not Now, When?*, not just for myself, but for my friends and family quite frequently.

A good friend of mine, Tom O'Lenic, had an idea for a book that he carried around in his brain for over twenty years. A Pittsburgh native, he had seen his city wrestle with a difficult period of deindustrialization transformation in the 1970s and '80s. Through it, though, Pittsburgh emerged as a glittering example of a New Economy city, whereas its Rust Belt cousins—like Detroit, Cleveland, and others—continue to struggle. In Tom's mind, the galvanizing thread that kept Pittsburgh working together toward a brighter future was rooted in the city's special relationship with its professional football team, the Pittsburgh Steelers.

Tom thought the story would be a great book, and he would talk about it almost endlessly with his wife and friends. I had heard his thesis a number of times. Finally, one day post-stem cell transplant, I asked—or maybe *told* Tom, as the case might be—"If not now, when?"

Answering the question for him, I told Tom there was no better time than the present and that I would help him. Soon thereafter, we started writing a manuscript, and less than two years later, we published *Immaculate: How the Steelers Saved Pittsburgh*, a book of which we're both incredibly proud.

I used my motto to act as a bit of a spur under Tom's saddle, and I lent my writing ability to Tom as a gift to see him through to completing what was a project of passion for him. That's what good friends do, after all, isn't it? Help our friends when they need it?

In turn, Tom gave a gift back to me, suggesting we donate all of our writers' proceeds from *Immaculate* to the University of Pittsburgh

Medical Center Hillman Cancer Center and the Multiple Myeloma Research Foundation.

If Not Now, When? led me to record music and release it on streaming platforms, both with the Chronic Padres and as a solo artist. But it has led not just to completing tasks on the deliverable of inanimate objects. Every bit as important, it's led me to rekindle relationships in my expansive list of contacts.

Tomorrow is not promised, so reach out and touch someone, right?

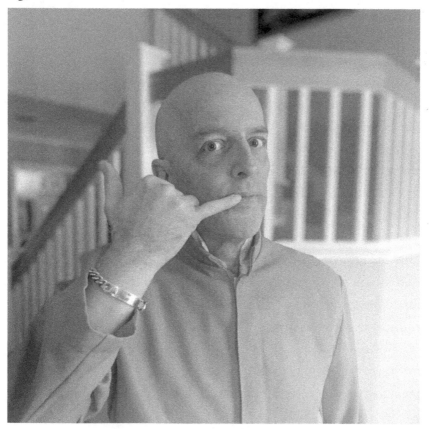

While follicly challenged, the author took advantage of his lemons to make lemonade.
(Photo courtesy of Lori Hartjen)

Speaking of which, *Tomorrow Is Not Promised* just might be coming to the back of a Chronic Padres T-shirt in the near future, right after *Stay Calm and Rock On.*

The motto/rallying cry I use most often is *Punch Today in the Face.* I just love that idea of letting today know you were here, using it up, and sending it back to the barn, ridden hard and put up wet. And then, just as I'm dozing off to sleep at night, giving tomorrow a nudge, pointing to it, and telling it I'm coming for it next.

Years ago, as an organizational development consultant at Sony, I frequently facilitated training sessions. One of my favorite courses was the Franklin Covey time management course, *What Matters Most.*

A very memorable part of the course was a timeline exercise that participants performed just for themselves, not to share with the rest of the group. A simple, introspective exercise, it was incredibly powerful to a great many, including me.

Let's do it together, right now, the two of us. On a stretch of blank paper, draw a horizontal line. On the far left of that line, place a short, vertical tick mark—that mark represents your birth. Then, on the far right of the line, place another short, vertical tick mark. You guessed it; that represents your death.

Now comes the eye-opening part. On that line, that representative timeline of your life on Earth, place a third vertical tick mark on the spot where you think you are now. The length of the line to the left of that third vertical mark is history. That space to the right represents what you think is yet to come.

For a great many of us, that third and final tick mark is a lot further to the right than we might have intuitively thought ahead of the exercise.

Looking at your timeline, how do you feel? Are you surprised at all? Can you feel that fire of urgency burning a bit hotter in your belly? I know I sure can.

If not now, when? Go out and punch today in the face!

For me, I need my mottos, as they're a reminder to resist falling into the taken-for-granted habits of yesteryear. Sometimes, and more often than I like, I need to snap out of a tendency to settle for comfort. Too often, at least for me, comfort is a disguise under which taking time and relationships for granted lurks in hiding, ready to ambush.

I genuinely fear slipping back into taking time and relationships for granted. It's a hard habit to break, maybe because it was formed by fifty-plus years of taking too much for granted, too often. I need my reminders.

Those reminders act as catalysts for proactive action on my part. Those actions, in turn, lead to me feeling good, leaving me feeling higher degrees of both satisfaction and inner peace. And how is that not good?

So I ask you, friend and reader, "Who's buried in your particular 'taken for granted' tomb?"

#PunchTodayInTheFace

Chapter 13

TAKING THE STEPS TO PHYSICAL RECOVERY, ONE AT A TIME

After being discharged from the hospital, Lori and I spent one more night in our home away from home, the Residence Inn in Menlo Park, where we packed up everything we had brought with us, from clothes to a toaster oven. The next morning, we checked out and beelined our way to our home in Pleasanton.

It was fantastic to be home, particularly for the Thanksgiving holiday that was being kicked off the very next week. I still had next to nothing with regard to an immune system, but I didn't let that stop us from going to my bandmate Scott's home for an hour or so on Thanksgiving. I was very much the weird, outlier house guest, hairless and wearing a mask while walking around—not my HEPA filter mask but just a regular, old mask. Or, rather, what would become regular in just a few short months, when the COVID-19 pandemic reared its ugly head in the United States.

I was feeling better and better, seemingly stronger every day. During a follow-up visit with Dr. Weng, he encouraged me not to look at my strength and my general feeling on a day-to-day basis. Instead, for the first month or two, he suggested I look at my health from a week-over-week perspective. Simply, was this week better than last week? For me, each week was definitely better than the one previous.

By mid-December, I was comfortable in my skin and with my bald head, and I had zero reservations about going out in public. It was great to meet up with friends to share holiday cheer, and I was most grateful for being able to spend the Christmas holidays with my family.

Then we ushered in 2020, and the post-holiday blues set in. I struggled mentally and emotionally. Physically, I felt pretty good, certainly considering what I had experienced just a couple of months before. My medical team warned me that my recovery from the stem cell transplant procedure could take six to twelve months. However, by the end of February 2020, I felt really good, and I believed I was getting close to being fully recovered.

I had regained most of the weight I had lost during the transplant process, and I felt fairly strong. I wasn't lifting weights or anything, and I know I was nowhere near the physical strength levels I had six months before. But I was plenty strong enough to complete normal, everyday activities both at home and at work.

Oh, sure, by the end of the work week, I was fatigued. And I hadn't really tested myself physically, but I had been consistent with light exercise. On a Saturday in late February, on my mother's birthday, I got out and took a solo hike up on the ridge, about five miles, the first half of which was uphill. My body responded well, both during the hike and afterward. Physically, I was on my way back to normal, or at least a new normal. But mentally and emotionally, I was struggling with an overall malaise.

I wasn't unhappy. I still enjoyed days of smiles and laughter, and I was blessed to be constantly encouraged by my circle of supportive friends and loving family. It's just that I wasn't my typical positive self.

As I approached the one-year anniversary of my initial diagnosis, I had the blues, and I thought it was kind of weird because passing the one-year mark should be ushering in all sorts of positive feelings. I mean, c'mon, it had been a heck of a year!

One year before, my bone marrow had been ninety percent cancerous. Five months later, it had been chipped down to less than five percent. Then, my stem cell transplant had knocked the level of cancer in my body to as low a level as it was ever going to get.

I felt as though I should have been skipping down to the bakery to pick up a cake.

Instead, I celebrated the first anniversary of my multiple myeloma diagnosis by undergoing a PET scan. Oddly enough, we didn't have any celebration planned. The one-year anniversary date of my diagnosis was just another day in the week that ended in a Y.

I don't know, maybe you don't celebrate your cancer diagnosis day, at least not with the same gusto and bravado you celebrate a wedding anniversary or a birthday. Still, a year is a logical milestone on the path of life, and there was a lot to look back on and acknowledge, particularly the gratitude I felt—and still feel—toward so many and their supportive actions.

I know I could have used the mental pick-me-up of having a celebration—just to break me out of my bluesy malaise. A few days after my one-year anniversary, I published a blog post that dove into my anniversary and my mental state of mind. It was a good catharsis, and it served to snap me out of my funk.

The blog post also prompted me to run out and buy a cake so Lori and I could have a belated celebration to mark the milestone.

My malaise wasn't some post-holiday season funk that so many experience. The timing was just coincidental—the blues were coming; it just happened to be as the calendar worked its way into 2020.

No, the root of my mental and emotional state was grounded in being post-transplant. I had been put through a bit of a wringer with the entire process, and in the end, I still had cancer. Through everything Lori and I had endured up to that point in time, I was still a cancer patient with an unknown future.

And hey, guess what? I had always had an unknown future, right? We *all* have unknown futures. But I would argue there's something more blissful, naively blissful, in pondering a diagnosis-free future.

However, in thinking further about my case of the blues, I knew my uncertain future wasn't the source. It might have been a contributing factor, but I had the persisting thought it was more a symptom than anything else. I set off to dig deeper through my mental and emotional self to uncover the true root.

One root was my resumption of active treatment for multiple myeloma. I can't remember the exact date that I resumed treatment, but I believe it was sometime in February 2020, just three months after my "extra birthday."

My maintenance treatment began with another daily dose of Revlimid, albeit a 10 mg capsule, as opposed to the 25 mg capsules I took leading up to my transplant. Additionally, I started receiving Velcade injections again, this time on a schedule of once every two weeks as opposed to my previous weekly schedule.

Initially, although I couldn't articulate it mentally for a while, I viewed the resumption of active treatment as a definitive step backward. Before my transplant, there was hope I could go a long time, maybe even over a year, with no maintenance medication whatsoever.

Now, here it was, less than three months after having my transplant, and I was right back to being somewhat tethered to the infusion clinic and getting poked in the abdomen.

My maintenance treatment led me to ask, "Why did I even undergo the stem cell transplant?" My medical team advised me that my transplant was absolutely the correct thing to do, and the timing of it was spot on. However, with the aggressive nature of my particular multiple myeloma, coupled with my relatively young age and my body's favorable response to my initial induction treatment, a maintenance regimen made the most sense. The advancements in treatment for multiple myeloma and the longitudinal studies that have accompanied them led my doctors to prescribe this maintenance program. The bottom line was, with an early start on a maintenance regimen, I should live longer.

Fine-tuning my maintenance doses, however, proved to be a bit problematic. We were simply too aggressive at first. I think my initial maintenance dose of Revlimid came on a four-week on, one-week off cycle. Coupled with the Velcade injections, my blood values plummeted.

With Dr. Weng off on sabbatical, my follow-up visits related to my transplant were being handled by Dr. Surbhi Sidana, who is trained in advanced hematology, with an emphasis on myeloma, amyloidosis, and dysproteinemia disorders. She was adamant about suggesting a degree of restraint in my maintenance medication, emphasizing that we were "in a marathon, not a sprint."

My blood values were all over the place, up and down, but definitely trending down. For one scheduled infusion, my neutrophils were below the threshold for treatment, resulting in a postponement of that week's Velcade injection, and only contributing to shading my mood a darker blue.

Finally, after going through a period of trial and error, Dr. Raj and I settled into a routine that kept the Velcade infusion every two weeks at a dosage of 2.78 mg mixed to 1.11 mL and limited the daily 10 mg Revlimid doses to a cycle of three weeks on and two weeks off.

Sounds simple enough, no? Try explaining that schedule to a specialty pharmacy and insurance system that has processes in place that are based on calendar months.

As of the writing of this chapter (April 2023), I'm still on that medication regimen and schedule. And I still battle low blood cell counts. My white blood cell count is almost always below the minimum of 3.3. About twice a year, it pops up above that threshold, and when it does, it sure feels good.

My neutrophils are usually above the low end of the range, 1.2, and have been above the minimum threshold of 1.0 to allow for every scheduled treatment to go through as planned. Sometimes just by the thinnest of margins, though. Like my white cell counts, on the occasions when I have neutrophils seemingly to spare, I smile and feel good about it.

While I had been walking a bit during my stem cell transplant and immediately afterward, it was much more *activity*—getting up and about and moving around—as opposed to *exercise*. There wasn't really a conditioning aspect to it, and I certainly wouldn't have referred to it as training.

I was taking a leisurely walk every other day or so, and I would guess my walking totaled six or seven miles a week.

As an athlete, I've always been goal-oriented. Exercising and working out becomes training if I have a goal to work toward, be it a game, a season, a race, or another event. For me, training for an event or a goal is much more motivating. Working toward a tangible outcome helps keep me going, and keeps me growing.

On the bicycle, I used to set mileage goals as stepping stones to some real buster-type events, like the California AIDS Ride, a week-long, 575-mile trek from San Francisco to Los Angeles; the Ride around Mt. Rainier in One Day (RAMROD), a 155-mile torture-fest that goes over three mountain passes; and the Mt. Diablo Challenge, a one-hour uphill romp that always took me to my very limit.

In late-February 2020, three months after my transplant, I saw a Facebook post from my friend and former coworker, Stacey Hames, about her progress toward her two year-long goals. First, there was a one-year, no-beer campaign. Then there was the 1,000-mile challenge, a quest to walk at least 1,000 miles in a year.

Well, truthfully, the no beer for a year was a non-starter for me. That wasn't likely to happen, no matter the health consequences. But the 1,000-mile challenge? Now, that was something I could rally around.

Walking 1,000 miles in a calendar year requires you to knock out an average of 2.74 miles a day, each and every day. That doesn't sound bad, right? It's a realistic goal. That is, if you can commit yourself to walking every day.

Skipping days, however, can be problematic. Skip one day, for instance, and the next day you have to walk 5.48 miles just to stay on pace. Skip two days, and . . . well, you get the idea. At those distances, things get a bit more difficult.

For my 2020 1,000-mile challenge, I started off on the wrong foot, so to speak. You see, I didn't see Stacy's post until late February. I had some making up to do—a lot of skipped days for which to atone!

There was no time for me to watch the grass grow. If I wanted to walk 1,000 miles, I had to get started working on it, one step, literally, at a time.

The first thing I needed to do was to increase my cadence of walking. No more days off for a long, long time. Second, I needed to ramp up my daily mileage considerably. Since I was just starting to track my mileage, I had to go over my daily quota of 2.74 miles to make up for the fifty or so days that had already elapsed in the year.

By mid-March, I had felt a real increase in my stamina, as it came back to me fairly quickly, thanks in large part to all those deposits I had placed in the pain bank during my decades of bike riding.

For the non-cyclist reader, there's a folklore-ish quality in the cycling world about suffering and a rider's ability to tolerate extreme effort when needed, like attacking on an uphill climb or extending oneself for a long period during a time trial. All those extensive, many times uncomfortable or downright painful, training rides come to be viewed as figurative deposits in the bank, providing a balance of conditioning for one to withdraw when a future ride or race calls for it.

For me, I made my withdrawals and saw an almost immediate improvement in my stamina. I had the strength to not only do my daily walking mileage and then some but also the ability to repeat the process the next day, and the next, and the next, and so on.

Of course, the COVID-19 pandemic hit the United States hard in the middle of March 2020. The impact was swift, in almost every facet of our daily lives. On my professional front, I lost my job. On my personal front, I lost the Multiple Myeloma Research Foundation's annual San Francisco 5K run and walk.

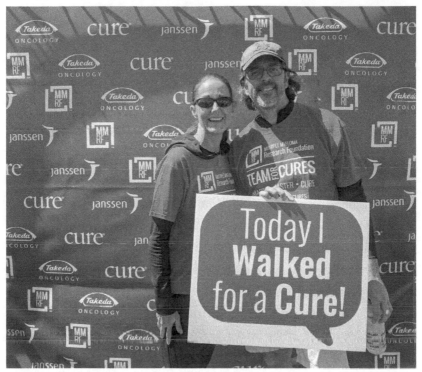

Donna Truex (l) and the author at the annual MMRF 5K in San Francisco, in March 2019, just three weeks after the author's multiple myeloma diagnosis. (Photo courtesy of Paul Truex)

The year before, I had attended the event with both Paul and Donna, and it was really uplifting for me. I had been diagnosed less than three weeks before, and my head was still spinning. To see all those patients and caregivers together on a glorious, sunny Sunday morning was inspiring. I had looked forward to participating again, to reunite with my extended community for another day of public defiance against our shared disease.

Since the event was scrubbed for our collective public health, I walked my own 5K, or 3.1 miles. And I kept walking.

By August 24, I had made up my deficit from starting the challenge late. That milestone, to be on a 2.74-mile-a-day pace, had been a huge carrot dangling in front of me for six months. However, that just got me level to the pace I needed to be on that date, at that snapshot of time. There was still work to be done.

Finally, on December 11, I crossed the 1,000-mile threshold and achieved my goal. In a nice piece of symmetry, I achieved my goal on Stacy's birthday. I ended 2020 with 1,047 miles walked and four pretty worn-out pairs of shoes.

Those weren't miles calculated on steps, where my tally would include walks through the grocery store and other similar activities. Rather, those miles were tracked on my activity app—I use the free version of the Runkeeper app—and were very much exercise activities designed to sustain an elevated heart rate. How successful I was is debatable, for my app showed that my average pace for those 1,047 miles was a rather pedestrian 16:18 per mile.

So, being a goal-oriented individual, I looked to surpass 2020's metrics in 2021. I wanted more miles and at a quicker pace. That year, I passed 1,000 miles on November 8, and true to form, I kept walking. In 2021, I walked 1,151.62 miles—and, yes, those 0.62 miles are important for me to track—at an average pace of 15:17 per mile.

Motivated by successfully hitting and surpassing my goals the previous two years, I set out in 2022 to break my marks for both miles and pace. On October 29, I broke the 1,000-mile mark. Accomplishing it by the end of October was a goal, and it meant that I averaged over one hundred miles a month. For the entire year, I finished with 1,160.18 miles walked at an average pace of 15:08.

It seems now, though, that I've walked myself into a bit of a pickle. I'm a believer that if I'm not improving, I'm regressing; if I'm not growing, I'm dying. Here I am, a year shy of my sixtieth birthday, wondering if I can hit walking totals in 2023 that exceed those reached in 2022. With a week left in April, I'm at 388.04 miles at a 15:01 pace.

Knock on wood that I keep the pace up!

Leaving my neighborhood, there are two general directions to take during my daily walks. One takes me through a nearby business park and a pleasant trail that runs along an arroyo. A bonus on that trail is an old parcourse.

Now, I'm not referring to parkour, the activity or sport of rapidly moving through an area, typically an urban environment, and negotiating obstacles as efficiently as possible by running and jumping. No, parcourses are generally remnants of the 1970s and 1980s, where jogging trails would sport various stations every 300 to 400 meters or so where exercisers could do prescribed calisthenics and work various muscle groups—usually shoulders, chest, abdominals, thighs, and calves.

What's great about my local parcourse is that it has a station with pull-up bars.

I've always thought pull-ups were the ultimate indicator of functional strength. The exercise is simple: with your arms extended, pull up your own body weight.

The thing is, I've never been great at pull-ups. I could always manage a few, but I've never been the guy to rip out a quick set of ten or more. Plus, I've had a variety of shoulder injuries in the past that have kept me from building on my pull-up repetition count. As soon as I start to make progress with increasing my repetitions, an injury tends to curtail my ability to work out.

Wanting to up my overall physical strength, the parcourse pull-up bars, being so ideally positioned, called out to me. So two or three times a week, I'd pause my tracking app and jump up and grab the bar.

I can't remember how many reps I pulled the first day—my guess would be two or three. But it at least gave me a baseline to work with, a daily minimum for me to shoot for every time my walks took me on that course.

Over the summer of 2020, I slowly improved. It got to the point where I was ripping nine or ten reps on my first set. With multiple sets, I'd work to get twenty-five reps in before continuing with my walk.

Like with almost everything in life, I've found improvements in physical conditioning are not the result of the work I do occasionally, but rather the work I do *consistently*. Daily exercise requires time, and sometimes it's difficult for us to carve out time in our busy days. But that time devoted to physical activity is an investment in ourselves, and who better to invest in than ourselves? Finding time most every day to be active is a non-negotiable for me. There are the rare occasions I'm limited, like days that require me to travel, for instance. But those days are few and far between.

Exercise is important for us all, but I think it's even more so for those who endure chronic health issues. I know, for me, physical activity—of which walking is just one part—makes me feel strong and active and, most importantly, does *not* make me feel like I'm sick and frail.

When I feel strong, I feel powerful, like nothing can stop me. That helps my mental and emotional state tremendously. It also gives me the energy to go to the market and source nutritious foods, prepare and eat healthy meals, and, in turn, fuel tomorrow's physical activities. It's all interrelated, an interlocking system of physical, mental, emotional, and spiritual health.

My daily walks are quite meditative. My walks allow me time to reflect, create, and recreate. Getting out and listening to the birds, breathing in fresh air, and just soaking up some of the outside world and nature I so often take for granted does wonders for my daily disposition.

Come on, won't you join me in the 1,000-mile walking challenge? Give it a try for just one month, or 83.3 miles. Then look back on how you feel, both physically and mentally. You might just discover an activity you'll make part of your daily routine from now on. And while you're at it, take a shot at that pull-up bar too.

My physical strength and stamina was not the only thing that needed to be rebuilt after my stem cell transplant. Another very important reconstruction job entailed that of my immune system.

As you'll recall, the chemotherapy doses completely destroyed my bone marrow, and with it, my immune system. The reintroduction of my stem cells was a hard reset. That day, November 5, was called my "extra birthday" by my medical team for a reason. While my body was fifty-five years old, my immune system was that of a newborn baby. And you know what that means—childhood immunizations.

Yes, that's right. Patients who undergo a stem cell transplant have to start all over with their immunizations, and I mean *all over*, from the very first one. In fact, the vaccinations are given in pediatric doses.

I figured the best way to get pediatric doses of immunizations was to go to a family doctor, which pretty much means a pediatrician. I liked my pediatrician so much that she's now my primary care physician. For each appointment, I am by far the biggest kid sitting in her waiting room.

At the one-year mark after my transplant, I started receiving my immunizations, and they involved repeated injections into my shoulders. There were multiple injections given each visit, and there were a series of immunizations that required me to go back every month.

I mean, there are a lot of doctor visits and injections to go through. No wonder most children don't like going to the doctor's office. And, by the way, whatever happened to the old sugar cube immunization, I think for polio? I remember that pleasant surprise of a treatment from my first go-around with childhood immunizations. Alas, the second time around, I wasn't as lucky.

Again, my mother would not recognize the guy who now calmly sits and takes syringe after syringe without a peep. It's still not my favorite activity, but it's got to be done, so grin and bear it I do.

After twenty-five months, I received my final measles, mumps, and rubella (MMR) booster, marking the completion of my schedule of vaccines. While it didn't clear me to go to preschool or anywhere else, it did provide me with a degree of comfort in navigating a world that was deep into a global pandemic.

Chapter 14

A DIFFERENT SLANT ON BEING DISABLED

On March 7, 2020, I performed with my bandmate Scott in our first Chronic Padres gig of the year. Being a perfect winery and brewery band, at least in our minds, it was fitting that we performed at BoaVentura de Caires winery in the Livermore wine valley. It was a cold and drizzly day, so we performed inside their big red barn. And while the crowd was relatively light because of the weather, they were attentive and fun.

It was a great morale boost for me. Together, Scott and I had planned a robust gig schedule for the spring, summer, and fall of 2019. Then came my diagnosis, and our plans went up in flames.

Not to be deterred, we were setting out to make 2020 different! We followed up the winery gig with a three-hour set at a restaurant/bar in downtown Pleasanton the very next Saturday, March 14. During breaks and after the show, there was a lot of talk going around about the novel coronavirus and the possibility that our downtown establishments might have to close.

The next day, I shared pictures from the gig with my family in our group text channel, and my sister, Ruth, the emergency room physician, immediately wrote back and told me I was stupid and irresponsible for being out in a crowd. She may not have used those words exactly, but if she didn't, she used words close enough that the message certainly hit home.

Going through my stem cell transplant, I was nervous about catching even the slightest bug. In the immediate months afterward, I was cautious, washing my hands more than I ever had. With my compromised immune system, I was fearful of catching even the most minor of infections.

But the idea of performing music again was so uplifting for me. It made me feel like a return to normalcy, to the time before my diagnosis. I didn't want to listen to the news of the quickly spreading coronavirus. Up to that point in time, mid-March, I had ignored the news, sort of like an ostrich burying its head in the sand.

Ruth's rather matter-of-fact message woke me up. The global COVID-19 pandemic was sweeping over us all, and as an immuno-compromised individual, I was particularly vulnerable.

It didn't take long for the dominoes to fall for so many of us. A week after Scott and I performed that second gig, I became a professional casualty of the pandemic, being laid off from work. In response, I became a full-time professional musician. Unfortunately, there was no place to play!

Needing groceries and health care—note, having a chronic health condition is Expensive, with a capital *E*, and, in many cases, a lot more uppercase letters following that first *E*—I was thrust into the job market, seeking my next opportunity.

The job application process can be an eye-opening, introspective experience if you allow it. I always find creating a resume and associated cover letters to be an anxious period, one filled with self-doubt about whether I'm telling the best stories, the ones that will seize the attention of both recruiter and hiring manager and present myself as a candidate that absolutely must be spoken with during their selection processes.

Each and every call back I *don't* receive leaves me wondering what I can do to improve upon my story.

Then there are the demographic questions at the end of almost every application—gender affiliation, ethnicity and race, veteran status, and a new one for me, personally: disability.

On employment applications, disabilities are listed as one or more of the following:

- Blindness
- Deafness
- Cancer
- Diabetes
- Epilepsy
- Autism
- Cerebral palsy
- HIV/AIDS
- Schizophrenia
- Muscular dystrophy
- Bipolar disorder
- Major depression
- Multiple sclerosis (MS)
- Missing limbs or partially missing limbs
- Post-traumatic stress disorder (PTSD)
- Obsessive-compulsive disorder
- Impairments requiring the use of a wheelchair
- Intellectual disability (previously called mental retardation) [note: their words, not mine]

There I am, clocking in at number three on the list—cancer. With my multiple myeloma, my selection to the question is now, "Yes, I have (or have had) a disability."

Kind of a strange word, *disability*. It's a noun, defined as "a physical or mental condition that limits a person's movements, senses, or activities; a disadvantage or handicap, especially one imposed or recognized by the law."

Now, I know I'm a bit late to this party. People have been fighting the stigma of "disabled" for decades. I've learned over the years to think of those afflicted individuals as being "differently abled" as opposed to "disabled." They have abilities. It's just sometimes some of them have to do things differently.

Filling out application after application had me thinking about my particular situation. In fact, I still think about it.

I'm fifty-nine years old, stand six feet, one inch tall, and weigh about 200 pounds when I stand on the scales every two weeks at the infusion center, fully clothed but minus shoes. I have a resting pulse rate between fifty-two and fifty-eight beats per minute, and that's not my pulse when I wake up in the morning but my pulse when I'm sitting in a chair at the infusion center and having my vital signs taken.

My blood pressure is in the 120-something over mid- to low-sixties. In addition to walking about three miles a day at slightly over a fifteen-minute-a-mile pace, I also lift weights and do a variety of flexibility exercises. My first set at the pull-up bar is ten on a good day, nine on a bad one.

And, oh yeah, I have multiple myeloma.

I have to believe that if I didn't have cancer, I'd be one of the more healthy individuals in any workplace. Try as I might to forget about it, I do have cancer, and it requires some reasonable accommodations. I need to visit my infusion center every two weeks for a Velcade injection in my abdomen. Plus, I have other doctors' appointments from time to time, although a great many of them have transitioned to video calls.

But disabled or disadvantaged? I don't feel disabled in the slightest. I feel quite comfortable stacking up what I can do with anybody, any age, any time, any place, in any and everything I have a right to stick my nose into and compete. I mean, I'm not going to out-engineer an engineer, but I sure as heck will out-write a writer and out-market a marketer.

At the end of the day, "I have (or have had) a disability," but I'm not disabled. Far from it. I'm fully abled, and I kick butt every day. After all, I'm a cancer patient who's fighting cancer—kicking butt is what we do day in and day out, without fail.

Chapter 15

SCANXIETY

have learned much from my support group meetings. I certainly feel as though I have taken much more than I have given, although I suspect most of the group members feel that way.

Group is an odd, collective relationship. We used to meet in person, upstairs in the very same facility where I receive my Velcade infusion treatments. The COVID-19 pandemic changed that, of course. Now our meetings are held virtually, via Zoom. With a little luck, we'll resume in-person meetings soon.

Currently, my attendance is spotty, hitting maybe one out of three—working a full-time job makes a 2:00 p.m. Tuesday afternoon group meeting difficult to attend. I went to my first group meeting within a couple of weeks of my initial diagnosis. I had never been to a group meeting of any type before, but I figured if there was ever a good time to get started, a cancer diagnosis felt like the right time.

For six months, I probably attended four out of every five meetings. Some of my peers were there every week. Others, maybe half of the meetings. Every once in a while, new patients would give group a try, some returning for more meetings, others deciding it wasn't for them.

Over time, we developed trusting relationships, although they tend, for me, to just take place during those two-hour periods every week. I only know the surname of one of the members, Mike Brown, a fellow multiple myeloma patient who was diagnosed about two weeks before me. I think my first group meeting was his second meeting.

I knew the surnames of two other individuals from group. Tony Leavens was a big guy, with a loud, booming voice. He used to attend with his wife—she was the one who actually convinced him to give group a try, as she felt Tony was overflowing with anger after his diagnosis of colon cancer. Tony used group to help deal with his cancer treatment but mostly used it to come to grips with his grandson's battle with cancer.

I bumped into Tony and his wife once in downtown Pleasanton. Lori and I were out for a drink, and sure enough, there was Tony and his wife, along with a circle of their friends. He came over and introduced himself to Lori, and we chatted a bit. He shared that he was excited about having someone in group who liked to do things he liked to do, like go downtown and enjoy a nice glass of bourbon. Or two.

It wasn't long after that I received an email with Tony's name in the subject line. Those are the absolute worst emails to receive. The email notified those of us on the distribution list that Tony had passed away because of an infection related to his chemotherapy port or PICC line (peripherally inserted central catheter).

Tony's death was a crushing blow to me. He was the first person to pass away since I had joined the group, and in my mind, Tony wasn't even ill. Sure, he had cancer, but he was to all appearances strong and vibrant. He and his wife were just about to go on a well-deserved cruise. I was left in shock.

Nancy Little was another long-time group member, someone who had participated in group for years before I joined. She, too, passed away unexpectedly—at least unexpectedly to all of us—from complications arising from one of her chemotherapy treatments.

Both deaths shook me to the core. As if I needed any reminders, their deaths were further evidence of the fragility of life, particularly those lives of patients dealing with serious health issues.

Perhaps I don't learn surnames, and don't bring group into my life outside of our weekly meeting, because I subconsciously fear loss. Well, now that I've written it, it's not subconscious anymore, now is it? Actually, it just seems ridiculous. Note to self: Get over yourself and embrace the human existence; develop those interpersonal relationships and grow, helping others along the way when there's an opportunity.

Okay, so now I've got some acknowledgments and apologies to make to the group, and a good place to start is with Gloria. Gloria, last name currently unknown to me, is a neighbor of mine. Seriously. Across the street and four houses down. Typical of modern suburban life for so many of us, it took a cancer patient support group for us to meet, despite the fact we're neighbors.

Then, there's another Nancy, a patient who has been in the group for much longer than me. Nancy recently checked off an item from her bucket list by learning to fly an airplane. She took her lessons from the husband of a third group member, a lymphoma patient whose first name I can't even remember. As I wrote, acknowledgments and apologies—plural.

Two of my most lasting takeaways from group have been dangling carrots and the foreboding uncertainty that surrounds medical tests.

Dangling carrots are those big milestones set off in short- and mid-term calendars that provide motivation to persevere and fight. Of course, they're different for each patient. Some are eyeing a child's graduation or wedding; others are earmarking the calendar for an international trip. Dangling carrots keep patients focused on today and tomorrow, and less on yesterday.

For me, those dangling carrots slotted right into my training regimen. Instead of a bike race, now I've got a music festival, the Indy 500, the publication of this book, and my daughter Olivia's wedding. There's always something to work toward, and so I feel myself always working, and working on moving toward, forward, and not backward.

Another big topic common to many group sessions is planned tests. Cancer patients are regularly tested. For example, I have a blood test taken every two weeks prior to treatment. If my blood values are high enough—particularly my neutrophil count—then I receive treatment. Conversely, if they're not high enough, treatment is postponed and then the wondering and worrying get ratcheted to an entirely new level.

Aside from routine tests, there are periodically more sophisticated tests, like magnetic resonance imaging (MRIs), PET scans, bone density scans, and a host of others. Leading up to a test, there tend to be weeks, even months, of foreboding worry. Simply, we all worry the test results will be poor, indicating we've taken a step backward in our fight against cancer.

Those foreboding feelings are heightened right after the test is completed and the wait for results begins. Some patients impatiently check their electronic medical records to see if results have been released. Others, like me, just wait to talk to their doctors at their next regularly scheduled appointment.

At group, that foreboding feeling awaiting tests and their results is called "scanxiety." It's this pessimistic, unfounded feeling that one's getting worse, or that we're setting ourselves up for bad news. In many ways, it's a self-protective defense mechanism, where we expect the worst and hope for the best. And I can tell you, scanxiety is real, at least for me.

Oddly, it didn't start that way. Going through the long road to a diagnosis, I was rather matter-of-fact about it. Part of it, I think, was a feeling of "it is what it is," that it was something beyond my control, so why bother worrying about conjecture and all the possibilities? However, a big part of my rather lax attitude, perhaps the biggest part of it, was undoubtedly denial—surely there's a reasonable, non-lethal, treatable explanation for my initial test results. Oh, and my secondary test results as well. And of course, the tertiary test results. You get the idea.

Then, related to testing, came my natural inclination to think more along the lines of, "I can hardly wait for this test and see how great I'm doing."

However, during my induction therapy, I started experiencing my first bouts of scanxiety with my weekly blood tests ahead of my treatments. Just a simple glance at the values on my CBC would give an indication of whether I was positively responding to treatment. Fortunately, within a week or two, I saw a marked improvement in my red blood count, to the point where I was no longer anemic. We couldn't be certain, of course, not without another bone marrow biopsy, but the test results allowed my medical team and me to logically assume that some of the cancer cells had been eliminated, thereby making more room for healthy bone marrow and its production of more red blood cells.

With my positive response to my induction treatments, my level of scanxiety was reduced right up until my stem cell transplant began. First, there was the daily testing of my blood leading up to the apheresis stage. Were my daily Neupogen injections working with my Cytoxan dose to coax my stem cells out of my marrow and into my bloodstream?

My scanxiety ramped up after apheresis and the recovery period, when I stepped into the second phase of the transplant process. After my stem cells were reintroduced, it was a waiting game to see if engraftment occurred. Engraftment usually occurs between ten and fourteen days. That's a long time to wait, and those days are filled with anxiety.

Waiting for engraftment, I was looking at daily blood values that were basically zero. No immune system whatsoever. And the lack of an immune system, as worrying as that can be to someone who has a few hypochondriac-like tendencies, was the least of my worries. What if I never engraft?

You know, I don't know the answer to that question. I'm rather hoping I never have to ask that question aloud.

Over time, my sense of scanxiety has grown. It's not crippling or anything like that, but it's certainly a stronger feeling and one I definitely work on reconciling.

Multiple myeloma is, at this point in time, incurable. While I have responded well to treatment, I know I still have cancer in my body. And while my cancer is currently undetectable in my blood tests, scanxiety rears its ugly head in wondering just exactly how long that will last. When will be the first sign that I am slipping back into the grasp of multiple myeloma?

A quick online search on multiple myeloma shows an average life expectancy of about five years after diagnosis. Well, I'm working to go well above average. However, I'm fully aware that as I type this sentence, I'm ten short months away from my five-year mark.

And wouldn't you know it? I have another PET scan scheduled in three weeks.

What will those results bring? Will this be the test result that denotes a marked decline in my health?

About six weeks ago in group, Jennifer—again, last name unknown (hey, I'm working on it!)—went into more detail about her ongoing bout with anxiety. Over the last year, she frequently brought up her crippling anxiety and her struggles to find the right medications and dosages to alleviate it. She never mentioned what she was anxious about, only that she had anxiety. Like a lot of patients, she was at first a bit reluctant to go too deep into specifics, like she was the only one who had a particular issue and the rest of us wouldn't fully understand.

It's funny how we sometimes feel that way. Then, over time, we come to the realization that a great many of us feel the same way, and deal with similar, if not the exact same, issues.

Anyway, Jennifer finally felt comfortable enough to share that her anxiety centered on an obsession with time. Jennifer works full-time as a surgical nurse, so her days are filled, not only with activities but also with rather time-sensitive appointments too. As a result, Jennifer found herself constantly obsessing about time. Did she have enough time to complete one activity before she had to start another?

For Jennifer, the obsession with time doesn't limit itself to work. It's everything in her life. For example, she regularly worries if she has enough time to cook dinner. Jennifer recognizes the root of her time obsession quite probably lies in her lung cancer diagnosis. Like all of us, she doesn't know what tomorrow might bring.

Jennifer's sharing stuck with me for a number of weeks. I kept thinking back on it, ruminating, letting it all marinate into my conscious and subconscious mind, and I couldn't help but feel this little itch that seemed to want some scratching.

Maybe I'm a slow learner; I don't know. But about three weeks after that group session, it finally dawned on me that I'm rather fixated on time myself. I'm not at the point where I need anti-anxiety medication, or at least I don't think I am. But I am most definitely focused on time, sometimes obsessively so.

You know I like my rallying cries. I'm always thinking of some sort of motto that motivates me to take action and, naturally, looks good on the back of a Chronic Padres band T-shirt. "Punch Today in the Face" is one of them, and it's entirely about making the most out of the gift that today is for each and every one of us. With each tick of the clock, today starts to slip away from us. So let's make those ticks count.

But what if I try too hard to make each and every one of those ticks count? Is it possible to be so fixated on time and accomplishing tasks that I overlook the simple joy of living in the present? You know, the whole idea of "taking time to smell the roses."

Punching today in the face has led me to publish a book and record songs, among other things. I certainly don't take time for granted nearly as much as I did before. But in focusing so much on accomplishing tasks, do I make myself more vulnerable to backsliding into taking my relationships for granted?

Naturally, in thinking that, I immediately set out and made a lunch appointment with my dear friend, Beth Baptist. How much more task-oriented could I be when I make working on fostering relationships a rather inorganic task? I talked to Beth about it during our two-and-a-half-hour lunch out in the sun on a glorious Sunday afternoon. She advised me that I should look for ways to embrace the present and take a long, loving whiff of the roses.

I have a lot of work to do in that regard. Just six days later, I found myself driving back from the grocery store. I thought about what I had accomplished so far that day—a 4.15-mile walk, 1,000 words written in this manuscript, and my grocery shopping done for the week. I felt this fleeting moment of prideful satisfaction as I glanced at the clock in my car and saw that it read just 11:23 a.m.

Then I thought to myself, *would it be all right if it was 11:30 or 12:00 noon?* Dude, relax a little. Would it kill you to take a minute and chat up the guy behind the fish counter? Maybe take a pause on your walk and take a picture of that deer nibbling on the leaves of a tree?

Okay, so that last one would mess up my per-mile average pace, but I think you can read where this is going.

My personal obsession with time goes beyond tasks and includes what probably borders on the trivial, like aiming to drink at least a gallon of water by 1:00 p.m., knowing that if I can, I'll be at a pretty good pace for the day. An even better one is my obsession with successfully completing the daily Wordle puzzle before I get out of the bathroom in the morning.

The past several weeks, my coworkers and friends have probably grown tired of me discussing my peculiar fixation on time. However, it's been a positive revelation for me. I never, ever would have shared this much about me personally, even just a few short years ago. Now, I figure the best way to really explore ideas and feelings is to share them with others and see if I can talk them out a bit with them.

I get a strong sense that making the most of time is going to be one of my strongest-held values for the rest of my life. I just need to find a balance, one where I feel fulfilled and hold a strong sense of satisfaction and inner peace while being able to take deep breaths and appreciate this wonderful gift of life by just *being*.

As an undergraduate student at Eastern Kentucky University, we used to have a professor who was fond of saying, "Moderation is the key to life." In many ways, he was probably correct.

Then again, that mantra is a bit uninspiring, leaning more toward mediocrity than the truly memorable. I mean, use a simple standard distribution illustration, the familiar bell-shaped curve. Do I want to be moderate, right there in the middle, leaving myself possibly feeling "meh" about everything?

No, not at all, not me. I think I'd prefer to be on the outlier ends of the bell-shaped curve. I tend to not desire the mundane and the moderate, and instead gravitate toward the unique, the wonderful, and the exceptional. I want to squeeze every last drop out of a great many things, like sunrises and sunsets over the beach, clean mountain air, a perfectly brewed cappuccino, sitting with Lori in our big red Adirondack chairs, and enjoying Kenny Chesney summertime concerts with my daughter, Olivia. But I do recognize I don't need to squeeze in every little thing.

It's like my view on competition and winning or losing. When I'm asked whether I love to win or hate to lose, I respond with, "It depends." There are a great many things in which I don't care to compete at all. I couldn't care less if I win or lose, and it doesn't affect my self-worth, pride, or ego one bit. For instance, playing the card game Phase 10 with my family. I don't care where I place in the standings. I just care about being with my family.

Now, there are other areas where I love to win, one of which is in business. That's a non-negotiable. There can be only one winner in the race for the customer. Even finishing second in this race leaves one as only the first loser.

Revisiting that old Franklin Covey course I used to facilitate, there was an interesting video we used to show. In it, Stephen Covey, the author of *The 7 Habits of Highly Effective People*, brings a seminar attendee onto the stage, where she is presented with a transparent bucket half-filled with pea gravel. Next to the bucket lies big rocks with words painted on them, like "Vacation," "Big Project at Work," and the like. Her task is to put the important things in her life into the bucket, which represents her available time.

Sure enough, she can't fit in all the big rocks that are important to her. She leaves some important items out, and she even reluctantly trades items she had already placed in the bucket with those big rocks for which she absolutely, positively has to account. Despondent at her realization she can't do all she wants, she tosses her hands into the air and sighs.

Then, at the height of her despair, Covey brings out another transparent bucket of the same size. He tells her to approach the exercise in a completely opposite manner. Instead of starting with the little rocks in the bucket, a metaphor for all the minutiae in our lives, what would happen if she started with the big rocks?

Energized, she quickly starts stacking all her important big rocks into the new bucket. She puts in everything from her old bucket and adds those items that she previously couldn't fit. Then, Covey helps her pour all the little rocks from the first bucket into the second bucket.

By placing the big rocks first—those rocks that represented that which was most important to her—she was able to fit everything, both big and little rocks, into the second bucket. In the second bucket, the little rocks worked themselves into all the empty spaces surrounding the big rocks.

So I have a time thing. Maybe a thing that goes so far as being a time anxiety thing. Recognizing it, I think I'm perhaps nipping it in the bud, not allowing it to grow and fester into something problematic.

My entire thought progression on the topic, including all the discussions I've had with friends, centers on balance. There are things I want to accomplish, roles I play in my life for which I am accountable. I need to get things done. I just need to pick and choose. Go all-in on those things I find most important and take a complete pass on those I find unimportant. Oh, and maybe give myself a break every once in a while.

At fifty-nine years of age, I'm still a work in progress. But progressing, I am. For the record, today, another Saturday, among other things, I walked 4.16 miles, wrote over 1,500 words, completed my weekly grocery shopping, and noticed it was 12:04 p.m. on my short drive home from the store.

Ha! Who says you can't teach an old dog new tricks?

Chapter 16

PERCEPTION AND A NEW REALITY

You've undoubtedly seen those mind-bending images, where you look at a picture and see one thing, while someone else views the exact same picture and sees something else entirely. Two of the most widely shared images are one that depicts, depending on your perception, either a beautiful young woman or an ornery-looking witch, while another shows two men arguing over the number of rectangular images they see, one seeing five, the other seven (some versions have it three versus four).

With respect to the two women, I tend to see the younger woman. In fact, even knowing that image well, having viewed it on so many occasions through schooling and my career, I have trouble finding the older woman—it always takes me a few seconds.

I tend to gravitate toward seeing one image. Others, including you, might see the other. And since our perception is our reality, we're both "correct."

The weird thing is, people being people, we spend an enormous amount of time and energy trying to convince those with differing perceptions that they should adopt our perceptions. We tend to steadfastly believe that our perception, our personal reality, is correct, and all others, with their personal realities they hold so strongly, are incorrect.

My, how quickly we jump from perception to judgment, don't you think? Personally, I don't know if this rush to judgment has ever been worse in our society than it is today.

With all our access to information through technology, we think we're smarter. Unfortunately, technology has also made many of us lazier. We have a lot of access to information, but we only consume and digest a small portion, just a fraction. Let's face facts, folks; we tend to be headline readers and scanners. That deep dive exposé on a subject, that effort to become truly knowledgeable about a situation or an issue, is quickly going the route of the dodo.

We think we might be smarter, but we're usually only tricking ourselves. Most of us are not smarter, of course. In fact, a very sound argument can be made that we are, collectively, not as smart as we once were. We read what we want to read, watch what we want to watch, listen to what we want to listen. What we *want*, not what we *need*.

Part of that is human nature. When we're pushed, particularly when we're pushed for time, we tend to settle on what's comfortable and easiest. When looking for comfort and ease, technology is there to serve, but it comes at the expense of knowledge.

As consumers of information, we are fed a steady diet of what media networks and platforms think interests us most. If you click on conspiracy theory stories, you'll get fed a steady stream of conspiracy theory stories going forward. Your online news streams and feeds are curated to show you topics you've already read and viewed, again and again, and again. Click on another of those related stories, and the cycle perpetuates.

If you haven't seen *The Social Dilemma*, the 2020 docudrama where Silicon Valley experts sound warnings on the dangerous impact of social networking and how large technology and data companies manipulate and influence all of us, I highly recommend it.

Our individual perceptions on so many matters are reinforced for the simple reason that there is big money to be made on feeding us the information we want—again, not need—to confirm how we already feel. In 2023, in the United States, one of the major news networks settled a legal case for almost one billion dollars after knowingly reporting false news.

Why did they act in a manner so antithetical to the basic tenets of journalism? They did so because they wanted to cater to the hot-button interests of a majority of their viewers, enticing them to continue watching, knowing all along the higher the viewership, the more money the network could make through advertisements.

As written often in this book, when I was first diagnosed with cancer, it was a wake-up call for me a much needed one. I, like I'm sure so many others living their lives, was guilty of taking too much for granted. I took relationships for granted, and I took time for granted. I took tomorrow, next week, next month, next year, and even the next decades, plural, for granted.

Heck, I was going to live forever. And my relationships, aspirations, and dreams would still be there when I eventually got around to them.

Now, I knew better at the time, at least intellectually, but I pushed that aside, emotionally, because I didn't want to make the effort. Or perhaps I was ill-equipped in my ability to effectively handle emotional topics in the first place, to rectify it.

My diagnosis changed me a lot. It hasn't changed everything completely. I'm certainly a work in progress. I still live teetering in denial, dipping my toes, and, to be honest, much more at times into the deep pool of denial. But I also spend much more time as a realist, recognizing when I take things that are important to me for granted. When I recognize that, I try to be proactive and positive, and do something about it.

After all, if not now, when?

My cancer diagnosis has changed my perspective on pretty much everything, and for that change in perspective, I feel fortunate. I'm not quite there in thinking I was fortunate for my diagnosis, of course. But there have been positive ramifications.

My life is fuller now. I have additional roles, each of them with a purpose. I still have all the former roles I had, but now I've added patient community and patient caregiver advocate roles, and I find each of them rewarding. Plus, I've benefited from having a revised perspective on perception itself.

With my changing perspective, I've adjusted what means most to me, and what's truly important. Where do I want to spend my time, with whom, and with what? Conversely, where do I not want to spend my time?

I actively avoid spending time around negative energy. I refuse to go down the rabbit hole of spiraling despair, either in conversation, in reading, or in watching.

It's not that I avoid bad news. I'm just not going to feed on it, regurgitate it, and repeat that over and over again. What I look to do is acknowledge the news as living in the "so what" category and think more about the actions necessary to answer, "Now what?"

Negative energy is not exclusive only to bad news. Negative energy can often be found circulating around individual people, including those who are closest to us.

My personal and professional networks contain individuals who hold a wide variety of thoughts and opinions, all based on their individual perceptions that, in turn, form their realities. Naturally, I see it a lot in the cancer patient community.

Some patients will discover a vitamin, mineral, or some other nutrient, organic or heavily processed, and be absolutely convinced it is making them healthier. They quickly hop on the proverbial soapbox and tell me and others we should follow their lead.

Usually, they're seeking to help. Sometimes, they're seeking safety in numbers, as if more people are doing the same thing they're doing, then they must be doing something right. Then there are the few who just absolutely want to shove their remedy down your throat.

Others will advocate for bypassing established medical advice based on something they've watched, read, or been told, whether it's from a medical doctor or not. Just yesterday, a fellow multiple myeloma patient went on about the dangers of "unnecessary" COVID-19 immunizations, swearing that not only would he not take another, but he won't ever get a common influenza vaccination, the annual flu shot.

I found his arguments rather odd. He, too, underwent a stem cell transplant, and in follow-up, he received his childhood immunizations. So, he's not anti-vaccination. He's just fervently against these particular vaccinations.

At this writing, I've had four COVID-19 immunizations, in addition to one dose of Evusheld, a combination of two human monoclonal antibodies targeted against the surface spike protein of SARS-CoV-2, and believed, at one point in time, to be effective in warding off infection in some patients.

It turned out Evusheld perhaps wasn't so effective. Oh well. I don't regret taking my dose. I took that dose, as well as my four COVID-19 immunizations, because my doctors advised me to receive them. I trust my doctors. The only reason I'm typing this sentence right now is because of them, not in spite of them.

Of course, I'm not advocating blindly following one doctor's suggested prescriptive remedy. Gather your facts from a variety of trusted sources and specialists, and make your best-informed decision.

Note key words, like "facts," "trusted sources and specialists," and "best-informed decision." We should do it for our health. And we should do it for the nightly news too.

I respect the right of my fellow patients to have their perceptions, especially if they differ from mine. Who knows? I might learn something valuable from them simply by listening to understand. Plus, I don't even mind too much if they push a little, just a little, to try to change my perception. I need to remain flexible and open. I need to listen a heck of a lot more than I talk. Not only do I learn more, but I also find myself in healthier relationships.

Now, back to that negative energy.

I have friends who love to argue and debate, endlessly trying to convince others to adopt their points of view, their perception on an issue. Ultimately, I think they prefer the estranged relationship to any other form of relationship. As a result, those connections of mine have, over time, inched more toward acquaintances and further away from friends.

There's no judgment there from my side. It just is what it is. Over time, we grow closer to some, while, at the same time, we grow further apart from others.

One of my acquaintances recently shared with me that I had changed, and it was said with intonation that the change was not for the positive. Well, first things first; I have changed, absolutely and unquestionably. If my diagnosis alone hadn't changed me, I'd be internally tone-deaf. And I warn you all, in an ever-changing world, if you are not changing, or at least open to change, you're probably being left behind.

I have changed much over the course of my life, but my values, which drive my behaviors, haven't changed dramatically. Those values, instilled in me early by my parents and my community, continue to form the foundation for not only my behavior but also my beliefs and perceptions—my reality.

I've actually gone through the exercise of labeling my values. They are, in a very particular order that sometimes dictates the decisions I make: family, friends, fun, fitness, education, and challenge. Those values have remained relatively consistent for nearly twenty-five years, although each of them has changed throughout that time.

You'll notice there's no value of work, for example. Well, yes and no. I don't value work, per se, but I certainly do work, and I'm blessed to be able to do so. But work, for me, is challenging and educational, so it caters to those two values. I look at a great many coworkers as friends, and I enjoy working and working with them. Again, consistent with my values.

Thus, while work, my profession, isn't a value for me, the right job with the right people can be very consistent with my values. My self-identity is not tied to my career. I've pivoted many times in my career, seeking jobs and a career that better fit my values, which I believe forms my identity.

All this brings me back to the beginning of this chapter and our perceptions and the individual realities they form.

Remember that timeline of our lives from earlier? The inescapable truth is we're all moving toward the right. Not a single one of us is promised tomorrow, and at the same time, today is coming to a close with each passing second. Do we really want to spend our time on the relatively trivial and damage the relationships with the ones we care about the most?

Spurred on by both media and technology, it seems society today is focused on broadcasting our perceptions, beliefs, and, on rare occasions, our values, all the while shouting down any conflicting perceptions, beliefs, and values of others. Everyone seems to be yelling argumentatively, but no one appears to be listening with an open mind, evaluating objective data, and making informed decisions. We're all correct, and everyone who disagrees is wrong. We're not very civil in the manners with which we communicate those opinions.

Some of our bickering just seems so counterintuitive and illogical. Look, for instance, at the single-issue voter, that person who will vote for a candidate for public office based entirely on the candidate's position on one issue. That lack of balance is potentially dangerous, don't you think? That must be one heckuva single issue.

I have friends who will push a point of view on a single issue to the point of dangerously threatening the foundation of our friendship. Some of those friendships have ended, and moved to the acquaintance classification, because of our differing views on an issue.

Those friendships didn't dissolve because of my actions. Well, other than my action to not acquiesce and adopt their point of view. Rather, they moved the relationship from friend to acquaintance because they could not reconcile the fact that I had a different point of view on one singular issue.

I miss those friends. I've told them our differing views, our differing perceptions, didn't change my love for them. Some of them have heard that, and we've moved forward. Others don't seem to have heard me, and we've moved on.

Still, I can't help but think if we could all take a step back from bombastic headlines and statements, listen attentively to other viewpoints, think for ourselves, and, most importantly, act civilly, with love, kindness, and compassion, we'd be closer. We'd be closer as friends. We'd be closer as citizens. We'd be closer as people.

A diagnosis of a critical health issue is one sure-fire way to change one's perceptions about a lot of things. Frankly, it becomes a case where a patient might begin to live like he or she is dying.

If you knew you were dying, would you set out to do anything differently?

I know now, post-diagnosis, that I have done things differently and that I will likely continue to do so. It doesn't make what I did before more right or more wrong, just different. And different works for me.

Cancer has changed my perspective on a great many things. However, I know that my perspective isn't shared by everyone, and I'm okay with that.

I recently had a conversation with a friend who is in his mid-fifties. Thinking he hadn't had a colonoscopy yet, I asked him if he had, in fact, had one. He replied that he hadn't, and he wasn't planning on having one anytime soon, as there is no family history of colorectal cancer.

I asked him to reconsider, and he said he would. But he said it in a way that was clear that he wasn't going to make an appointment and that he was just moving on with the conversation, hoping I'd quit nagging him.

I love him, and I care for him. I'll gently nudge him again in a few months. At the end of the day, though, I know he's got his one life, and he's going to live it the way he feels best, and I respect that. Likewise, I know he respects me and the way I live my life.

My hope for us all is that we understand each other and our perceptions. We need to back off the strong feelings that one is "right" and the other is "wrong." In the vast majority of the situations, those differing perceptions are just that—they're different.

I've got an incurable blood cancer. Do I really want to spend my time needlessly arguing with others so they will eventually adopt my beliefs? Or do I want to spend my time having others repeatedly try to convince me to adopt their perceptions, particularly on issues that don't really make a difference to me, my values, and those I care about the most? My answer to both questions is a resounding, "No."

You might be different. You go be you, and be the best you that you can be. That won't change my love for you.

I just ask that you respect me trying to be the best me I can be. I'm hopeful your love for me also won't change as a result.

Chapter 17

THAT TERMINAL CONDITION WE CALL "LIFE"

Just a couple of pages ago, I posed the question, "If you knew you were dying, would you set out to do anything differently?" It's the idea, and perhaps even the ideal, of living like you're dying.

Of course, we're all dying. We all have that terminal condition we call "life." We're all in this together, and no one gets out alive.

Truthfully, I've never been fond of the idea of dying. Since I was a young child, I've known, intellectually, that I won't live forever. However, I've never accepted, emotionally, that I was going to die.

Note the differences in my language. I know I won't live forever. But I never thought I was going to die. Yeah, it's semantics. However, I'm a writer, and if words don't matter to me, to whom will they matter?

I've never been one to ponder death, at least not for very long. It's not that I'm scared to die. Oh, believe me, I am absolutely scared to die. The idea terrifies me. But no, I don't think much about dying because I've always been caught up in the act of living. I absolutely love, L-O-V-E love, living life.

I even like the bad days, the days when nothing seems to go right. Really, I do. So much so, I've had intellectual and emotional blinders on my entire life as it relates to clinical depression and other mental health ailments. As a younger person, I couldn't contemplate those conditions; I just didn't understand.

I still don't understand depression nearly enough. Knowing those who have had treatment for their issues has helped, but on those occasions when they've shared with me, while I try to be empathetic, I don't really understand what it's like to walk even the shortest of steps in their shoes. It's almost unfathomable to me.

I've been extraordinarily blessed throughout my life, and I know that I have had things relatively easy. I certainly have not endured hardship after hardship, continuously stacked upon one another.

I mean, I grew up in a stable household, with both of my parents providing love, support, and encouragement. We weren't wealthy, not on my father's military salary, but we didn't want for much. We had plenty of food on the table. And when the time came to go to college, I didn't have to work to pay tuition, room, and board.

Just that alone gave me a huge head start during my first twenty-two years of life, and I'm extraordinarily grateful. I know a great many people who have had it more difficult than me. I've had some hardships along the way, but if I'm truthful with myself, I know a great many of them were self-inflicted.

A diagnosis of any serious medical condition, cancer certainly included among them, often brings a natural tendency to ask, "Why me?" Those thoughts sometimes pop into patients' minds, and they can be particularly counter-productive and self-destructive if allowed to fester and grow unchecked.

Heck, I'll admit it; sometimes those thoughts come flying into my head. I might come across someone who I know has a list of unhealthy vices longer than the length of my arms. Yet, I'm the one with an incurable cancer.

Why me?

I immediately kick myself into what I believe is a better thought, asking the better question, "Why not me?"

I also realize it's sometimes much more difficult for others to make that quick pivot, moving from "Why me?" to "Why not me?" Many times, those are people who find themselves fighting through one hardship after another, seemingly never gaining ground before something else comes along and slaps them back even further.

I recognize that I've been blessed many more times than not, and I'm eternally grateful. It's with tremendous gratitude that I know I'm not alone, that I'm unconditionally loved, that I'm gainfully employed, that I have health insurance and a sound financial foundation, and that I have . . . so much. I often feel my cup has runneth over.

We all have our limited time to grace the planet; the timeline exercise makes that abundantly clear to even those with the strongest sense of denial. A fact of our existence is that we all get something. Some of us even know what that "something" is, although I'm not certain that's a blessing or a curse.

I have multiple myeloma, a blood cancer. That's what I have now. No telling what else I might add to it down the line. Be that as it may, I'm working, day in and day out, on making multiple myeloma not be my "something."

Oh, sure, multiple myeloma may one day be curable. CAR-T (Chimeric Antigen Receptor) cell therapy is the latest, greatest medical advancement that shows promise. It's a treatment similar to my stem cell transplant.

In CAR-T cell therapy, T cells are first taken from a patient's blood. Then the gene for a special receptor that binds to a particular protein on the patient's multiple myeloma cells is added to the T cells in the laboratory. Large numbers of those T cells are then grown in the lab and reintroduced to the patient via infusion.

Maybe one day, if, or maybe when, as the case may be, my multiple myeloma climbs back to a magnitude that suggests I have relapsed, I'll be a candidate for CAR-T. But that's not something I think about much today.

Today, I think about fighting my cancer to the point that it's another "something" that I'll have to add to my fight card. If I succeed in fighting my multiple myeloma, I know there'll be something else to follow.

We all get something. It's part of the condition we call life. I'll fight one foe until I have to fight another.

Hey, why not me?

I've always been a fan of sunsets, much more so than sunrises. Primarily, it's because of when they occur. Sunrises come just a little too early for this guy. I mean, seriously, to catch a sunrise, you have to wake up before the sunrise or, at the very latest, the "crack of dawn."

No, for this guy, I've always gravitated toward sunsets. They simply fit into my daily schedule better. I've always been a bit of a night owl, anyway.

All of that is beginning to change as I get older. Changing quite dramatically, actually.

These days, a night owl, I am most certainly not. I am often in bed well before 10:00 p.m. Maybe once or twice a month is the exception. *Maybe.*

I typically read for about thirty minutes before shutting out the light and falling asleep pretty quickly. Despite the relatively early bedtime, I still don't make too many sunrises, even during daylight savings time.

Now, I'm actually in bed for a long time. With my busy days of working, writing, playing guitar, exercising, and all my other activities, coupled with my ongoing treatment, I'm well worn out by sunset, and certainly by 9:00 or 10:00. I usually get up after 7:00 a.m. On those occasional luxuriously extravagant mornings, I might awake a few minutes past 8:00 a.m.

Well, that was before Lori and I brought home Quinn, our Goldendoodle puppy. Quinn usually begins to stir at 6:30 a.m. Still, I need the time, the sleep, to ward off fatigue and allow me to give my best in my fight against cancer.

I'd like to get my eyes on more sunrises, though. I like the metaphor. The sunrise is the beginning of the day, and each day is full of opportunities. Some of those opportunities will be presented to me. Others, I might have to create for myself. Either way, the day is a blank page, ready for me to write, paint, or otherwise make my own.

What will I do today to leave my mark? What will help me fulfill my purpose(s) and deliver feelings of inner peace and satisfaction?

Today is a new day, and I'm blessed—we're all blessed—to have it. A cancer diagnosis shines a brighter light, like the rays of the sun, on the fact that tomorrow isn't promised. Given that, what are we going to do today?

🚶 🚶 🚶

I started writing this manuscript with the intent of telling my story, to possibly serve as a resource for those multiple myeloma patients and patient caregivers whose journeys and fights have just started. Over the past four-plus years, I've frequently had fellow patients reach out to me, asking about my experiences and to use me as a sounding board for not only their prescribed treatments, but for their personal thoughts and feelings as well.

Some patients are introduced to me by common friends. Others see me on social networking platforms and reach out. Still others have seen various videos and news stories to which I have had the pleasure of contributing.

Each time a patient reaches out to me, I am deeply humbled. It's an honor to listen to other multiple myeloma patients as they share their stories with me. I will always make myself available for patients and their caregivers, as not only is it my sincere pleasure, but I feel very much as though being a resource for my patient community has become my calling.

If there's a lasting impression I can impart, I would want it to be a simple, straightforward message. Cancer is not the entire identity of patients, nor is it the end, and I urge you to resist feeling it is. You, we, are all stronger than we know. More than that, we're even stronger together. Believe in yourself and know

> Cancer is not the entire identity of patients, nor is it the end, and I urge you to resist feeling it is.

deep in your heart there is not an illness or disability that can prevent any of us from having a dream and working determinedly to realize it.

At the same time, we all need to recognize the perils of potentially slipping into a state of toxic positivity, that induced pressure, either internally from ourselves or externally, from others, to display only positive emotions.

Cancer sucks, to put it bluntly. We, as patients and caregivers, get nowhere in the short- and mid-term by suppressing negative emotions and feelings that sprout up from our fights and journeys. Doing so can lead to unhealthy coping practices, and eventually crippling trauma. It's okay for us to feel what we feel.

However, we patients can't afford to wallow interminably with negative, though very real, emotions and feelings. Doing so prevents us from giving our best. Since cancer never takes a day off in attacking our bodies, we can't afford to give our fight anything less than our very best.

In the end, we all get something as this terminal condition we call life moves on. It's what we do after our diagnoses that matters most.

I hope my story, the narrative of my cancer fight thus far, sheds light on what other patients and caregivers might expect from their experiences with multiple myeloma. I also hope my story delivers hope and inspires others to fight back against cancer and live the full life they desire.

We all have our stories to share; thank you for allowing me to share mine. However, this isn't the end of my story, nor is it the end of yours. It might be more of the middle than the beginning, but it sure isn't the end.

I look forward to connecting personally with all of you. Together, let's help each other write the continuing chapters of the stories of our lives. Please consider joining this book's community by following its Facebook page at www.facebook.com/mymultiplemyeloma.

Take care, be well, and keep fighting.

Conclusion

NEXT STEPS

I t might be the end of the book, but it's far from the end of our collective fights and journeys. Tomorrow's a new day, a blank canvas full of opportunities for us to paint, and in a great many ways, tomorrow will be what we make it.

Together, let's make it great. After today, let's make a plan to punch tomorrow in the face too!

Whether you're a multiple myeloma patient, a patient of another cancer, a caregiver, or an ally, I do have some suggested and requested "next steps" for when you close the back cover of this book.

First, please consider joining *Me, Myself & My Multiple Myeloma's* online communities:

- Facebook (www.facebook.com/mymultiplemyeloma)
- Instagram (www.instagram.com/mymultiplemyeloma/)
- Reddit (www.reddit.com/r/mymultiplemyeloma/)

The intended purpose of those three communities is to share, back and forth, all those things that make us our complete, authentic selves. Our whole human experience—that which makes us, well, us. It's not only about being a cancer patient. Of that, cancer patients didn't exactly have a choice. Sure, it's a giant part of our lives, but if there's one hope I have for this entire book and its associated communities, it's that we, cancer patients, are so much more than just cancer patients. Cancer is a part of our identity. It's not and never will be our sole identity. Please consider joining and actively participating in our communities.

Additionally, please consider lending your voice to *The Patient Story* community, that community created by Stephanie Chuang, who so kindly provided the foreword to this book. All of you—patients, caregivers, and allies alike—have a voice and a story, and if you want to share it, I, for one, sure want to hear it. Together, we are strong.

In that light, continue to build your teams. As described earlier, choosing to share your diagnosis is a very personal decision, and there is no absolute right or wrong. What you choose is right for you. If you do share your diagnosis, seek to nurture those relationships with those that provide you strength. At the same time, you might want to consider limiting time around those who lessen your strength.

Whether you broadly share your diagnosis or that of someone you care for or care about, know you already have one member on your team. Me.

You can reach me at both rayhartjen@gmail.com or (925) 895-5441. If I can be of service to you and your loved ones, please let me know. Seriously.

Also, stay up-to-date on multiple myeloma by following along with news from the Multiple Myeloma Research Foundation (MMRF) and the International Myeloma Foundation (IMF). While somewhat slowed during the pandemic, advancements in the care and treatment of multiple myeloma continue at a dizzying pace. Educate yourself and discuss various treatment options with your medical team.

Finally, resist any temptation to give up or lose hope. As I wrote in the previous chapter, the reality is that we all get something at one point or another. Another reality is that our world is a better place with you in it.

Thank you for reading. Aside from sharing lives with my wife Lori and raising our two children, Oliva and Raymond, having you as a reader of my story is the biggest honor of my life. Thank you, again. Take care, be well, and punch today in the face!

Okay, one last "finally."

Finally, please consider leaving your authentic review at any bookseller's site. It's truly valuable for other potential readers.

ACKNOWLEDGMENTS

First and foremost, I would like to thank my wife of twenty-nine years, Lori. She's always been on "Team Ray," even on those occasions when I behave like maybe I shouldn't. And importantly, she never once wavered by my side as I underwent the tests that led to my multiple myeloma diagnosis and the many treatments that have followed.

Oh, Lori may have wavered at times by herself, or in the confidence of her friends. But, within earshot or view of me, she's remained my steady rock, providing unconditional love and empathetic compassion at every step and turn in our journey. She gives me strength daily, and I'm forever grateful.

Thank you, too, to our children, Olivia and Raymond. It's been the greatest honor of my life watching them grow to be the people they are and will be, and they inspire me daily to fight cancer with all my might.

I literally would not be where I am today without the love, generosity, and support of all the people I affectionately call "My Team." At the head of that list are Paul and Donna Truex, dear friends from the day I met them both way back in 2000. That list also includes, among many others, Tom and Chris Anne O'Lenic, Scott Sorochak, Cara Neff, Linda Mourer, Rob Manfredo, Jeff "Frog" Greer, Joe O'Loughlin, Steve Naiser, Rob Toth, Beth and Dave Baptist, Mike and Karmen Taft, Mark and Kim Olson, George and Kim Polites, Tom and Patty Powers, Joel and Kimba Warford, Dave and Marina Beadle, Kathy O'Loughlin, Jeff and Lori Christensen, George Frangos, Reece Keeler, Sean Haughian, Mike and Julie Bockover, Shareef and Renee Mahdavi, Brent Bockover, Randy and Fran Usedom, Bob and Patsy Zollars, Steve and Erin Iversen, Tim and Julie Morse, Teresa and John Held, Troy and Robin Treto, Rob and Dee Dee Nitzsche, Louise Matthews, Liz Almeida, Liz LeMaitre, Lou Bock, Scott Wells, Bram Sciammas, Matt Beadle, James Kozuch, Keiko Mitsunobu, Tyce and Tammy Whilhytle, Don and Jen Morrissey, Pat Walsh, Herb and Kathy Ritter, Don Errigo, Patti Polischuk, Taylor Truex, Kennedy Truex, Michael Kushner, Ken and Wendy Kushner, Fred and Lita Reiman, Erralyn Reiman, Wilet Tudela, Debra and Mike Mallie, Be'Anka Asholou, Drew Bush, Bridget Johns-Pavlopoulos, Darrell and Janis Emery, Mimi Black, and Nicola Lombardi.

Those I've missed, please accept my most sincere apology.

A big "THANKS" also goes out to my extended family, including my father, Ray, my mother Helen, and Ruth, Tom, Colleen, Noah, Audrey, Eli, and Sophie. Also, I want to add those who are no longer with us but who are never forgotten, including my mother, Irene, and Lori's mother, Alice.

I owe a continued debt of gratitude to Fran Carpentier, the "Godmother," who has ushered me through the entanglement of book publishing and promotion like only a renowned expert like she can.

Importantly, thank you to my editor, Cortney Donelson, whose feedback makes me a better writer while not crushing my fragile writer's ego, as well as the entire team over at Morgan James Publishing, including David Hancock, Naomi Chellis, Shannon Peters, and so many others. Without you all, this book never happens.

Finally, thank you all who are in the cancer patient, cancer patient provider, and cancer patient caregiver communities. My love for you all knows no bounds. And if I can ever be of service to you, please let me know at either rayhartjen@gmail.com or (925) 895-5441.

Take care all; be well.

#PunchTodayInTheFace

ABOUT THE WRITER

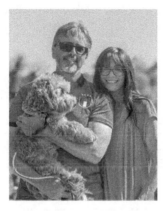

Ray Hartjen is a writer and musician who lives in Pleasanton, California, where he and his wife, Lori, raised their adult children, Olivia and Raymond.

In a professional career that has spanned parts of five decades, Ray has pivoted on many occasions, from investment banking to pharmaceuticals, from consumer electronics to SaaS software. One constant throughout his career path, however, has been storytelling.

In the past, Ray has been a frequent source for quotes from the national media on both the consumer electronics and retail industries. Additionally, as a contributor to a number of online outlets and platforms, including his rayhartjen.com site, he has spun his fair share of yarn on topics as far-ranging as sports—primarily football, hockey and auto racing—and business, particularly revenue team functions like sales and marketing. Ray's previous work includes being the coauthor of *Immaculate: How the Steelers Saved Pittsburgh*, published in 2022 by Morgan James Publishing and available at all major booksellers.

Diagnosed with multiple myeloma in March 2019, Ray is a cancer fighter every day of the week that ends in a 'y.' And, with the soundtrack of life playing continuously in his head, Ray also performs and records with his two-piece acoustic band, the Chronic Padres. A native of Texas, Ray holds an undergraduate degree from Eastern Kentucky University and an MBA from the University of Washington.

As one always to welcome a chat with others, especially fellow cancer patients, please feel free to connect with Ray at www.rayhartjen.com, on X/Twitter @RayHartjen, via email at rayhartjen@gmail.com, or via voice or text at (925) 895-5441.

ENDNOTES

1   "Why men get cancer more than women and how they can
    manage their risk." City of Hope. Feb. 9, 2022, https://www.
    cancercenter.com/community/blog/2022/02/men-and-can-
    cer-risk#:~:text=may%20know%20why.-,Doctors%20have%20
    known%20for%20decades%20that%20men%20are%20
    more%20likely,National%20Cancer%20Institute%20(NCI).

2   Katz, Rebecca, *The Cancer-Fighting Kitchen,* Second Edition:
    Nourishing, Big-Flavor Recipes for Cancer Treatment and
    Recovery; Ten Speed Press, February 14, 2017.

3   National Cancer Institute, https://www.cancer.gov/about-
    cancer/understanding/statistics#:~:text=Approximately%20
    39.5%25%20of%20men%20and,will%20die%20of%20
    the%20disease.

4   Nabissi, Massimo, et. al. "Cannabinoids Synergize with Carfil-
    zomib, Reducing Multiple Myeloma Cells Viability and Migra-
    tion." *Oncotarget 7,* no. 47 (2016). Accessed August 23, 2023,
    https://doi.org/10.18632/oncotarget.12721.

A free ebook edition is available with the purchase of this book.

To claim your free ebook edition:

1. Visit MorganJamesBOGO.com
2. Sign your name CLEARLY in the space
3. Complete the form and submit a photo of the entire copyright page
4. You or your friend can download the ebook to your preferred device

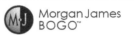

Morgan James BOGO™

A **FREE** ebook edition is available for you or a friend with the purchase of this print book.

_____

CLEARLY SIGN YOUR NAME ABOVE

Instructions to claim your free ebook edition:
1. Visit MorganJamesBOGO.com
2. Sign your name CLEARLY in the space above
3. Complete the form and submit a photo of this entire page
4. You or your friend can download the ebook to your preferred device

Print & Digital Together Forever.

Snap a photo

Free ebook

Read anywhere

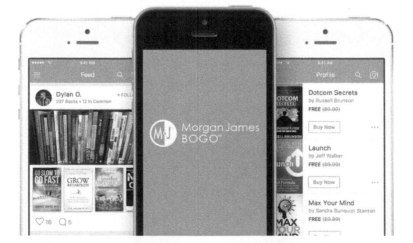

Printed in the USA
CPSIA information can be obtained
at www.ICGtesting.com
JSHW080923080624
64474JS00002B/23

9 781636 983349